MEMORY BANK FOR
NEONATAL
DRUGS

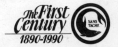

The First
Century
1890-1990

SANS TACHE

MEMORY BANK FOR NEONATAL DRUGS

Ellen-Marie Milan, RNC

Clinical Nurse III
Infant Special Care Center
University of California San Diego Medical Center
San Diego, California

Edward J. McFeely, BSPharm

Clinical Pharmacist, Pediatrics
Pharmacy Department
University of California San Diego Medical Center
San Diego, California

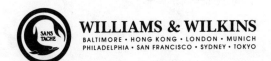

WILLIAMS & WILKINS
BALTIMORE · HONG KONG · LONDON · MUNICH
PHILADELPHIA · SAN FRANCISCO · SYDNEY · TOKYO

Editor: Susan M. Glover
Associate Editor: Marjorie Kidd Keating
Copy Editor: Barry Lerman
Designer: Norman W. Och
Illustration Planner: Lorraine Wrzosek
Production Coordinator: Adèle Boyd

Copyright © 1990
Williams & Wilkins
428 East Preston Street
Baltimore, Maryland 21202, USA

Accurate indications, adverse reactions, and dosage
schedules for drugs are provided in this book, but it is
possible that they may change. The reader is urged to
review the package information data of the manufacturers
of the medications mentioned.

Printed in the United States of America

Library of Congress Cataloging-in-Publication Data

Milan, Ellen-Marie.
    Memory bank for neonatal drugs / Ellen-Marie Milan,
Edward J. McFeely.
        p.   cm.
    Includes bibliographical references.
    ISBN 0-683-05976-9
    1. Pediatric pharmacology—Handbooks, manuals,
etc.   2. Drugs—Handbooks, manuals, etc.   3. Infants
(Newborn)—Diseases—Chemotherapy—Handbooks,
manuals, etc.   I. McFeely, Edward J.   II. Title.
    [DNLM: 1. Drug Therapy—in infancy & childhood—
handbooks.
2. Neonatology—handbooks.   WS 39 M637m]
RJ560.M45   1990
618.92′0061—dc20
DNLM/DLC   89-22678
for Library of Congress   CIP

                                        90 91 92 93 94
                        2   3   4   5   6   7   8   9   10

Preface

Providing drugs for newborns and infants is a hazardous undertaking. Immature clearance mechanisms, changing volume of distribution, extreme sensitivity to the effects and adverse effects of drugs all affect dosing recommendations. The dose that is correct for an infant today may be inappropriate for that same infant in two weeks.

The recommendations contained in this handbook are a compilation of data from many sources. In some instances, the literature offers conflicting recommendations. In those cases, we have recommended a dosing schedule that is both safe and effective. In other instances, we have advanced dosing recommendations that are a result of our clinical experience with careful pharmacokinetic monitoring of drug serum concentrations. The dosing guidelines recommended are for initial dosing of drugs. Dosing adjustments should be made based upon the infant's clinical response, laboratory parameters, and, where applicable, serum drug concentrations.

Some of the drugs included in this handbook are NOT approved by the Federal Drug Administration (FDA) for use in newborns and infants or even for use in children under the age of 12 years. Consult the manufacturer's product information (package insert) for FDA recommendations. There are occasions when drugs are used for non-FDA-approved indications if the practitioner believes that a drug will benefit an infant and that the benefits outweigh all the potential risks. The practitioner who uses a drug that is not approved for use in newborns and infants or for non-approved indications assumes liability for any therapeutic misadventures that may occur.

Before prescribing or administering any drug to an infant, the practitioner must be thoroughly familiar with the drug's indications, dose and dosing schedule, appropriate administration, effects, possible adverse effects and parameters to be monitored. Again, consult the manufacturer's product information.

Preface

Acknowledgments

We would like to thank Linda Levy, RNC, MSN, who brought our idea for an infant drug handbook to the attention of Carmen Germaine Warner, RN, MSN, FAAN. We thank Carmen for guidance in the early stages of our book, for finding a publisher, and for "pep talks" in the final stages. We also thank some special nurses, pharmacists, and physicians who reviewed our manuscript: Janine Dubina, RN, BBA; Lisa Sifford, RNC, BSN; Roberta Rehm, RNC, MSN; Philip O. Anderson, PharmD; James R. Lane, PharmD; William E. Murray, PharmD; Ron Coen, MD; and Fred Sherman, MD. A very special thanks to Lisa for making us both computer savvy. We also thank Susan Glover, RN, MSN, Editor for Nursing, and Margie Keating, Associate Editor, Williams & Wilkins for their encouragement and patience.

Contents

Preface   vii
Acknowledgments   ix

Chapter 1   **Administration of Drugs**   1
Intravenous Administration   1
Intermittent Injection   2
Intermittent Infusion   4
Continuous Infusion   5
Intramuscular Administration   6
Oral Administration   6
Rectal Administration   8
Subcutaneous Administration   8

Chapter 2   **Central Nervous System (CNS) Drugs**   10
Analgesics and Antipyretics   10
Acetaminophen   10
Analgesics and Sedatives   11
Chloral Hydrate   11
Fentanyl   13
Lorazepam (see Anticonvulsants)
Methadone   15
Morphine   18
Paregoric   20
Anticonvulsants   23
Clonazepam   23
Diazepam   25
Lorazepam   27
Phenobarbital   28

Phenytoin   33
Pyridoxine (Vitamin B$_6$)   36
Narcotic Antagonists   38
Naloxone   38
Stimulants   39
Aminophylline (Hydrous and
  Anhydrous)   39
Caffeine Citrate   42
Doxapram   44
Theophylline (Anhydrous)   46

Chapter 3   **Cardiovascular (CV) Drugs**   50
Antiarrhythmics   50
Digoxin (see Other CV Drugs)
Lidocaine   50
Phenytoin   53
Procainamide   56
Propranolol   59
Quinidine Sulfate   62

Antihypertensive Agents   65
Captopril   65
Hydralazine   68
Nitroprusside   70
Tolazoline   73

Sympathomimetics   76
Dobutamine   76
Dopamine   78
Epinephrine   82
Isoproterenol   85

Other CV Drugs   88
Alprostadil (PGE$_1$)   88
Atropine   91
Digoxin   93
Indomethacin   97

Chapter 4   **Neuromuscular (NM) Drugs**   102
Skeletal Muscle Relaxants   102
Atracurium   102
Pancuronium   104
Succinylcholine   107
Vecuronium   109

Chapter 5   **Renal Drugs**   113
Diuretics   113
Furosemide   113
Hydrochlorothiazide   116
Hydrochlorothiazide and
  Spironolactone   118
Spironolactone   120

Chapter 6   **Gastrointestinal (GI) Drugs**   123
Cimetidine   123
Metoclopramide   126
Ranitidine   129

Chapter 7   **Anti-Infectives**   132
Antibiotics   132
Aminoglycosides   132
  Amikacin   134
  Gentamicin   137
  Tobramycin   141
Cephalosporins   144
  Cefazolin   144
  Cefotaxime   146
  Ceftazidime   148
  Ceftriaxone   150
Penicillins   153
  Ampicillin   153
  Methicillin   156
  Nafcillin   158
  Penicillin G   161

        Piperacillin   164
Sulfonamides   167
   Sulfamethoxazole/Trimethoprim
   (SMX-TMP,
   Co-Trimoxazole)   167
Other Antibiotics   169
   Clindamycin   169
   Erythromycin   172
   Metronidazole   175
   Vancomycin   177

Antifungals   181
Amphotericin B   181
Flucytosine   184
Nystatin   186
Antivirals   188
Acyclovir   188
Ribavirin   190

Chapter 8   **Corticosteroids**   194
   Dexamethasone   195
   Hydrocortisone   198

Chapter 9   **Vitamins, Minerals, and
Electrolytes**   202
   Vitamins   202
   Folic Acid   202
   Vitamin D_2 (Ergocalciferol)   203
   Vitamin E (d,l-∂-Tocopherol)   206
   Vitamin K_1 (Phytonadione)   208
   Vitamins, Multiple   210

   Minerals   211
   Calcium Chloride 10%   211
   Calcium Glubionate   214
   Calcium Gluconate 10%   215
   Ferrous Sulfate   218

Electrolytes   221
   Arginine Hydrochloride   221
   Potassium Chloride   222
   Sodium Bicarbonate   227
   Sodium Chloride   229

Chapter 10   **Vaccines and Toxoids**   233
   Diphtheria and Tetanus Toxoids and
     Pertussis Vaccine Adsorbed
     (DTP)   233
   Hepatitis B Virus Vaccine Inactivated
     (Plasma-derived)   235
   Poliovirus Vaccines: Live Oral Trivalent
     (OPV) and Inactivated (IPV)   237

Chapter 11   **Miscellaneous Drugs**   241
   Normal Serum Albumin, Human 5%
     and 25%   241
   Heparin   243
   Hepatitis B Immune Globulin   246
   Hyaluronidase   247
   Immune Serum Globulin, Human
     (IV)   248
   Phentolamine   250
   Protamine   251
   Sodium Polystyrene Sulfonate   253
   Tromethamine   256
   Urokinase   257

Appendix A   **Cardiopulmonary Resuscitation**   262

Appendix B   **Electrocardiogram**   267

Appendix C   **Cardioversion and Defibrillation**   271

Appendix D   **Drug Information for Parents**   275
   Aldactazide   277
   Digoxin   279

Contents   **xv**

                  Furosemide   281
                  Phenobarbital   283
                  Theophylline   285

Appendix E   **Drugs in Breast Milk**   287

Appendix F   **Laboratory Values**   299

Appendix G   **Weights and Measures**   303

Appendix H   **Abbreviations**   306

Bibliography   308

Chapter 1

Administration of Drugs

Drugs are administered to infants via several routes: IV, IM, PO, PR, SQ, and inhalation.

Intravenous Administration

The most common route of drug administration in the sick infant is IV. The drug is administered directly into the blood, bypassing problems of absorption as with IM, SQ, PO, and PR routes. There is a more predictable onset of action and therapeutic serum concentrations are more rapidly achieved. Veins for the placement of peripheral catheters include the cephalic, basilic, and median antebrachial veins of the arm (Fig. 1.1), the great and small saphenous veins (and their branches) of the leg (Fig. 1.2), the supratrochlear and superficial temporal veins (and their branches) of the scalp (Fig. 1.3), and the veins on the dorsum of the hands and feet. Vessels for the placement of deep central catheters include the umbilical arteries and vein and the external jugular and subclavian veins. Intravenous drugs are administered by intermittent injection, intermittent infusion (e.g., aminoglycosides, amphotericin B, vancomycin), or continuous infusion (e.g., dopamine, dobutamine, PGE$_1$).

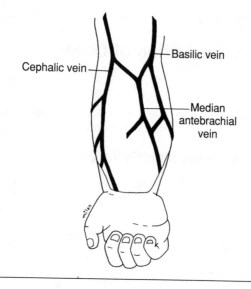

Cephalic vein

Basilic vein

Median
antebrachial
vein

Figure 1.1.

Intermittent Injection

Drugs injected intravenously should be administered as close to the infant as possible. Flashball injection sites are preferable over stopcocks and Y- and T-type injection devices, which contain dead space. The patency of the IV should be assessed prior to drug administration. Intravenous injection of concentrated drugs (high osmolality > 600 mOsm/kg

Memory Bank for Neonatal Drugs

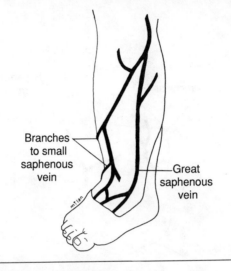

Branches to small saphenous vein

Great saphenous vein

Figure 1.2.

H₂O, e.g., digoxin, phenobarbital, phenytoin) can cause local irritation and phlebitis. Some drugs can cause tissue necrosis and sloughing when extravasation occurs (e.g., calcium, dopamine, nafcillin). Drugs are often diluted to decrease osmolality and potential for vein irritation. If drugs are to be diluted, a two-syringe technique should be used to avoid dilution errors (the measured drug dose is **added** to a syringe containing compatible diluent). The drug contained in the dead space (hub) of a syringe must be appreci-

Administration of Drugs

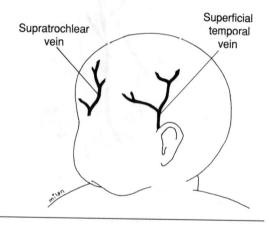

Supratrochlear vein

Superficial temporal vein

Figure 1.3.

ated; if not, the dose administered may be substantially larger than intended, resulting in "dilution intoxication." This will occur if the diluent is drawn into the syringe containing the drug dose or if the syringe containing the drug dose is flushed.

Intermittent Infusion

Intermittent infusions are used to administer drugs

that have a high potential for toxicity if administered too rapidly. Drugs administered by intermittent infusion are retrograded or piggybacked into an existing, compatible IV infusion or are infused via a heparin lock. Controlled infusion devices, such as syringe pumps, should be used for the administration of drugs by piggyback or heparin lock. Drugs should be retrograded or piggybacked as close to the infant as possible. Again, flashball injection sites are preferable over stopcocks and Y- and T-type injection devices, which contain dead space. Small bore IV tubing should be used for retrograding drugs. The small bore tubing promotes laminar flow of the drug, thus reducing mixing and adsorption of drug to the wall of the IV tubing. The final volume of the diluted drug for retrograde infusion is determined by the infant's IV rate and the desired infusion duration. The drug is retrograded by occluding the IV tubing at a point between the injection site and the infant to prevent the flow of drug to the infant when injected. The dose volume is then injected slowly into the IV tubing to prevent the drug from flowing too far up the tubing, thus prolonging the duration of the infusion. There are retrograde administration systems available on the market.

NOTE: Some drug may be lost if the IV setup is inadvertently changed prior to completion of the drug infusion.

Continuous Infusion

Continuous infusions are used to administer drugs that have a short duration of action. Serum drug concentration and therapeutic effect are constant. Controlled infusion devices, such as syringe pumps, should be used to ensure an accurate and steady infusion rate of potent drugs administered by continuous infusion (e.g., dopamine, dobutamine, nitroprusside).

Intramuscular Administration

In the term newborn, muscle tissue comprises about 25% of body weight (less in the preterm infant) as compared to 40% in the adult. Absorption of drugs administered IM depends on area blood flow and can vary among specific muscles. Drugs administered intramuscularly are slowly and less effectively absorbed in the infant because of poorly developed peripheral circulation and insufficient muscle mass. Conditions causing peripheral vasoconstriction (cold stress, asphyxia, shock) or poor circulation (edema) will delay absorption of drugs.

The vastus lateralis muscle, which is well developed at birth and free of major nerves or blood vessels, is used for IM administration of drugs in infants. The muscle can be isolated by pinching up the midanterolateral thigh. A short, small gauge needle (25G) should be used and inserted at a 90° angle. Gently aspirate back on the syringe before administration. Some drug may be lost due to leaking at the injection site. Administration of certain drugs can cause local irritation, induration, necrosis, and tissue sloughing.

Oral Administration

The second most common route of drug administration in the infant is PO. Absorption of drugs administered orally is influenced by drug formulation, presence of food in the GI tract, pH of stomach and intestines, gastric emptying time, digestive enzymes and bile salts, and intestinal motility. There is a less predictable onset of action, and therapeutic serum concentrations are more slowly achieved. Optimal absorption usually occurs if the drug is administered before feedings, but inactive ingredients (e.g., alcohol, preservatives, sugars) contained in PO preparations may be very irritating to the infant's GI tract, especially if administered on an empty stomach. Most PO drugs administered to infants are hyperosmolar (up to 20,000 mOsm/kg H_2O [FP]) and should be diluted to prevent potential GI irritation.

Oral drugs should be measured and administered by syringe or *calibrated* dropper for accuracy. Care should be taken to remove any air bubbles after drawing up the dose. When administering the medicine, the tip of the syringe or dropper should be placed between the infant's gums and cheeks or may be placed into the side of the infant's mouth, parallel to the nipple (breast or bottle), as the infant feeds. Because of the natural outward tongue thrust in infants, drugs may need to be retrieved from lips and chin and be refed. Oral drugs are often administered via an empty nipple or mixed with a *small* amount of formula or breast milk for administration via a nipple. Oral drugs should never be mixed with an entire feeding, since the infant may not take the entire feeding and thus receive only a partial dose of drug. Feeding tubes are used for administering PO drugs to small preterm infants and other infants with poor suck/swallow coordination. The site of drug absorption along the GI tract should be considered when PO drugs are administered by a gastric tube as opposed to a transpyloric tube in the duodenum or jejunum. Some drug may be lost with "spitting," vomiting, or the inadequate flushing of feeding tubes used to administer PO drugs.

Rectal Administration

Absorption of drugs administered PR is influenced by drug formulation (suppository vs liquid), presence of stool in the rectum, retention of the drug, and blood flow in the area. Rectal drug absorption is erratic and unpredictable. Administration involves the use of suppositories, which are usually too large for most small infants without adjusting their size (and thus the drug dose), or the use of "retention" enemas. Suppositories are gently inserted into the rectum, beyond both of the rectal sphincters, with the buttocks held together for 5–10 minutes after administration for optimal retention. Retention enemas are administered by gently inserting the tip of a soft lubricated tube into the infant's rectum and slowly infusing the drug while holding the infant's buttocks together during and after administration for 5–10 minutes for optimal retention. Some drug may be lost due to leaking from the rectum. Certain drugs can be irritating to the rectal mucosa.

Subcutaneous Administration

In the term newborn, subcutaneous tissue comprises about 16% of body weight (less in the preterm infant). Absorption of drugs administered SQ depends on area blood flow and can vary among specific subcutaneous tissues. Drugs administered subcutaneously are slowly and less effectively absorbed in the infant because of poorly developed peripheral circulation. Again, conditions causing peripheral vasoconstriction or poor circulation will delay absorption of drugs.

The anterior thigh, upper arm, and lower abdomen are used for SQ administration of drugs. The site can be isolated by picking up the subcutaneous layer in the desired area. A short, small gauge needle (25G) should be used and inserted at a 45° angle. Gently aspirate back on the syringe before administration. Some drug may be lost due to leaking at the injection site. Administration of certain drugs SQ can cause local irritation, induration, necrosis, and tissue sloughing. Administration sites should be rotated.

Chapter 2

Central Nervous System (CNS) Drugs

Analgesics and Antipyretics

Acetaminophen

Brand Names

Liquiprin, Panadol, Tempra, Tylenol, various

Forms

Drops 100 mg/ml, 120 mg/2.5 ml, 165 mg/5 ml (may contain propylene glycol and parabens).
Elixir 120 mg/5 ml, 160 mg/5 ml (may contain alcohol).
Suppository 120 mg, 125 mg.
Other concentrations of drops, elixirs, and suppositories are available.

Uses

Antipyretic (for fever).
Analgesic (for mild pain).

Dose

10–15 mg/kg/dose PO q 4–6 hours prn. Maximum daily dose is 65 mg/kg.

Pharmacokinetics

Rapidly and almost completely absorbed from the GI tract. Peak serum concentrations occur between 30–60 minutes. Half-life is 3.5 hours. Largely metabolized in the liver; 2–3% is excreted unchanged in the urine.

Cautions

Relatively nontoxic in therapeutic doses.

Use with caution in infants with G6PD deficiency or liver dysfunction.

Nursing Considerations

- Monitor infant's response to drug:
  - observe for signs of pain: irritability, restlessness, increased muscle tone, increased HR, RR, or BP.
  - monitor infant's temperature.
- Osmolality (Tylenol drops 100 mg/1 ml): 16,550 mOsm/kg H_2O (FP).

Analgesics and Sedatives

Chloral Hydrate

Brand Names

Various

Forms

Elixir 50 mg/ml, 100 mg/ml.
Suppository 325 mg.

Uses

Sedation/hypnotic.

Dose

Sedation: 25 mg/kg/dose PO, PR q 6 hours prn.
Hypnotic: 50 mg/kg/dose PO, PR.

Pharmacokinetics

Rapidly and well absorbed from the GI tract. Onset of action is 10–15 minutes after PO administration. Sedation is achieved within 15 minutes; sleep within 30–45 minutes. Metabolized in the liver to an active metabolite and excreted in the urine and a small amount in bile. Moderate plasma protein binding.

Cautions

Can cause vomiting and gastric or rectal irritation (depending on route). No analgesic effect (may cause excitement, not sedation, in infants with pain). Respiratory depression, hypotension, arrhythmias, and myocardial depression have been reported. Can cause laryngospasm if aspirated.

Use with caution in infants with heart disease or liver or kidney dysfunction.

Nursing Considerations

- Dilute drug or administer with feeding to decrease gastric irritation.
- Mix drug with cottonseed or olive oil for rectal administration. Administer rectally with lubricated tube. Hold buttocks together after rectal administration for optimal retention and absorption.
- Monitor HR, rhythm, BP, and respiratory effort.
- Assess infant's response to drug and duration of effect.

- Assess infant's need for sedation:
  - intolerance of handling and/or care.
  - agitation, restlessness, inconsolability.
  - change in vital signs (increased HR, RR, BP).
  - decreased TcO_2 and/or O_2 saturation, increased $TcCO_2$.
- Check stools and gastric residuals for occult blood.
- Monitor liver and kidney function.
- Protect drug from light.
- Osmolality (50 mg/ml elixir): 3620 mOsm/kg H_2O (FP).

Fentanyl

Brand Name

Sublimaze

Forms

Injection 50 mcg/ml.

Use

Analgesia (moderate to severe pain).
Sedation during mechanical ventilation of infant.

Dose

2–5 mcg/kg/dose IV q 2–4 hours prn.
2–3 mcg/kg/hour (maximum 5 mcg/kg/hour). Continuous IV infusion.

Pharmacokinetics

Onset of action is almost immediate. Duration of action is 30–60 minutes. Half-life is variable (1–15 hours). High degree of tissue binding and a highly variable disposition of drug in the neonate. Largely metabolized in the liver; 10% is excreted unchanged in the urine. Metabolism is dependent on liver blood flow and rate of release of drug from tissues. Highly plasma protein bound.

Cautions

Can cause bradycardia, hypotension, respiratory depression, decreased GI motility, vomiting, constipation, and urinary retention. Hypotension most likely to occur with inadequate or borderline blood volume. Rapid IV infusion can cause muscle rigidity, apnea, and seizures. Transient rebounds in serum levels can occur from minutes to hours after a dose due to release of drug from body tissues. Clearance can be delayed with abdominal distention due to decreased liver blood flow.

Dependence can occur with long-term use. Do not discontinue drug abruptly; can cause withdrawal symptoms.

Use with caution in infants with hypotension or liver dysfunction.

Use with caution in infants not receiving assisted ventilation.

Solution Compatibility

D5W, 0.9% NaCl, TPN.

Additive Compatibility

Atropine, heparin, metoclopramide.

Nursing Considerations

- Infuse slowly IV push over 5 minutes.
- Monitor HR, RR, and BP.
- Observe closely for respiratory depression due to potential for transient rebounds in serum levels.
- Monitor for adequate oxygenation and ventilation (blood gases, TcO_2, $TcCO_2$, O_2 saturation, color).
- Assess infant's response to drug and duration of effect.
- Reversal of drug effect: NALOXONE 0.01–0.02 mg/kg/dose. Repeat prn.
- Have means of assisted ventilation at bedside.
- Assess infant's need for sedation or analgesia:
  - intolerance of handling and/or care.
  - agitation, restlessness, inconsolability, increased muscle tone.
  - changes in vital signs (increased HR, RR, BP).
  - decreased TcO_2 and/or O_2 saturation, increased $TcCO_2$.
- Observe for signs of withdrawal after long-term use (tremors, irritability, hypertonia, high-pitched cry, vomiting, diarrhea, poor feeding, tachypnea).
- Observe for abdominal distention. Check for bowel sounds.
- Observe for urinary retention. Monitor urine output.
- Monitor liver function.
- Protect drug from light.

Methadone

Brand Names

Various

Forms

Oral solution 5 mg/5 ml (contains alcohol).
Other extemporaneously prepared forms are available.

Uses

Treatment of significant neonatal drug withdrawal
(SLEEPLESSNESS, progressive irritability, tremoring,
SEIZURES, POOR FEEDING, vomiting, diarrhea, and
WEIGHT LOSS or POOR WEIGHT GAIN or Neonatal
Abstinence Score $\geq$ 8 for 3 consecutive scores or for
an average of 3 consecutive scores). Used in infants
exposed to methadone with withdrawal refractory to
other drugs.

Dose

0.1–0.5 mg/kg/day PO q 12–24 hours. Adjust dose for
control of withdrawal symptoms.
Irritability and tremors should NOT be the only criteria
for initiating drug therapy or adjusting dose.
Maintain effective dose for 3–5 days before reducing
dose. Dose is reduced every 1–2 days as tolerated
(infant sleeps and feeds well and gains weight).
Duration of therapy is usually weeks to months.

Pharmacokinetics

Well absorbed from the GI tract. Half-life is 15–25
hours. Partially metabolized in the liver to active
metabolites and excreted in the urine and bile. Significant amounts of drug are excreted unchanged in the
urine.

Cautions

Can cause CNS depression, respiratory depression, decreased GI motility, vomiting, and constipation.

Do not discontinue drug abruptly; may precipitate withdrawal symptoms.

Use with caution in infants with liver or kidney dysfunction.

Drug Interactions

Phenytoin: effects of methadone may be decreased with possible precipitation of methadone withdrawal. Effect of interaction may occur up to several days after discontinuation of phenytoin.

Rifampin: effects of methadone may be decreased with possible precipitation of methadone withdrawal. Effect of interaction may occur up to several days after discontinuation of rifampin.

Nursing Considerations

- Onset of methadone withdrawal can present as late as 2–4 weeks after birth.
- Obtain urine for toxicology on suspected infants.
- Utilize Neonatal Abstinence Score to identify significant withdrawal. Observe infant for SLEEPLESSNESS, excessive or continuous high-pitched crying, hyperactivity, moderate to severe tremoring (especially when undisturbed), hypertonia, SEIZURES, POOR FEEDING, vomiting, diarrhea, and WEIGHT LOSS or POOR WEIGHT GAIN.
- Provide supportive treatment for withdrawal: swaddling, minimal noise and light, waterbed, pacifier, frequent feedings, holding and rocking.

- Monitor caloric intake and daily weights.
- During the initiation and maintenance of drug therapy: monitor HR, rhythm, rate and quality of respirations, color, perfusion, activity, tone, and level of consciousness.
- During reduction of drug therapy: observe for increased signs of withdrawal. Infant should continue to sleep and feed well and gain weight.
- Observe for abdominal distention and constipation.
- Administer with feeding.
- Protect drug from light.

NOTE: The oral dose is not the same as the IV dose. Only PO dosing/administration is considered in this manual.

Morphine

Brand Names

Various

Forms

Injection 2 mg/ml (may contain preservatives). Various other concentrations are available.

Uses

Analgesia (severe pain).
Sedation.

Dose

0.05–0.1 mg/kg/dose IV, IM q 4–6 hours prn.

Pharmacokinetics

Rapid onset of action after IV administration. Half-life and duration of action is 2–4 hours (may be longer in the preterm infant). Largely metabolized in the liver. Significant amounts of unchanged drug can be found in the urine of the neonate, along with metabolites. Some histamine release.

Cautions

Can cause respiratory depression, bradycardia and hypotension (due to histamine release), decreased GI motility, vomiting, constipation, and urinary retention. Rapid IV infusion can cause severe respiratory depression, hypotension, and circulatory collapse. Hypotension most likely to occur with inadequate or borderline blood volume.

Narcotics can cause respiratory depression severe enough to require assisted ventilation.

Dependence can occur with long-term use. Do not discontinue drug abruptly; may cause withdrawal symptoms.

Use with caution in infants with liver or kidney dysfunction.

Solution Compatibility

Dextrose-saline combinations, D5W, 0.45% NaCl, 0.9% NaCl, TPN.

Additive Compatibility

Atropine, dobutamine, metoclopramide, succinylcholine.

Additive Incompatibility

Aminophylline, heparin, methicillin, phenobarbital, phenytoin, sodium bicarbonate.

Nursing Considerations

- Infuse slowly IV push over 5 minutes.
- Monitor HR, RR, and BP.
- Monitor for adequate oxygenation and ventilation (blood gases, TcO_2, $TcCO_2$, O_2 saturation, color).
- Assess infant's response to drug and duration of effect.
- Reversal of drug effect: NALOXONE 0.01–0.02 mg/kg/dose. Repeat prn.
- Have means of assisted ventilation at bedside.
- Assess infant's need for sedation or analgesia:
  - intolerance of handling and/or care.
  - agitation, restlessness, crying, inconsolability, increased muscle tone.
  - changes in vital signs (increased HR, RR, BP).
  - decreased TcO_2 and/or O_2 saturation, increased $TcCO_2$.
- Observe for signs of withdrawal after long-term use (tremors, irritability, hypertonia, high-pitched cry, vomiting, diarrhea, poor feeding, tachypnea).
- Observe for abdominal distention. Check bowel sounds.
- Observe for urinary retention. Monitor urine output.
- Monitor liver and kidney function.
- Protect drug from light.

Paregoric

Brand Names

Various

Forms

Oral tincture 2 mg/5 ml (0.4 mg morphine equivalent/
ml). Contains camphor and benzoic acid.

Uses

Treatment of significant neonatal drug withdrawal
(SLEEPLESSNESS, progressive irritability, tremoring,
SEIZURES, POOR FEEDING, vomiting, diarrhea, and
WEIGHT LOSS or POOR WEIGHT GAIN or Neonatal
Abstinence Score ≥ 8 for 3 consecutive scores or for
an average of 3 consecutive scores). Used in infants
exposed to narcotics.

Dose

0.2–0.5 ml/dose (0.08–0.2 mg morphine equivalent)
PO q 3–4 hours.
Start with 0.2 ml. Increase 0.05 ml/dose until control of
withdrawal symptoms.
Irritability and tremors should NOT be the only criteria
for initiating drug therapy or adjusting dose.
Maintain effective dose for 3–5 days before reducing
dose. Dose is reduced every 1–2 days as tolerated
(infant sleeps and feeds well and gains weight).
Duration of therapy is usually 3–6 weeks.

Pharmacokinetics

Well absorbed from the GI tract. Half-life of morphine
is 2–4 hours (may be longer in the preterm infant).
Rapidly metabolized in the liver and excreted in the
urine and bile. Small amounts are excreted
unchanged in the urine.

Cautions

Can cause CNS depression, respiratory depression, decreased GI motility, vomiting, and constipation. Can also cause CNS stimulation and seizures due to camphor content and hyperbilirubinemia due to benzoic acid content.
Do not discontinue drug abruptly; may precipitate withdrawal symptoms.
Use with caution in infants with liver or kidney dysfunction.

Nursing Considerations

- Onset of withdrawal is shortly after birth to 2 weeks (usually within 72 hours).
- Obtain urine for toxicology on suspected infants.
- Utilize Neonatal Abstinence Score to identify significant withdrawal. Observe infant for SLEEPLESSNESS, excessive or continuous high-pitched crying, hyperactivity, moderate to severe tremoring (especially when undisturbed), hypertonia, SEIZURES, POOR FEEDING, vomiting, diarrhea, and WEIGHT LOSS or POOR WEIGHT GAIN.
- Provide supportive treatment for withdrawal: swaddling, minimal noise and light, waterbed, pacifier, frequent feedings, holding and rocking.
- Monitor caloric intake and daily weights.
- During the initiation and maintenance of drug therapy: monitor HR, rhythm, rate and quality of respirations, color, perfusion, activity, tone, and level of consciousness.
- During reduction of drug therapy: observe for

increased signs of withdrawal. Infant should continue to sleep and feed well and gain weight.
- Observe for abdominal distention and constipation.
- Acute overdose may be reversed with NALOXONE 0.01–0.02 mg/kg/dose. Repeat prn.
- Administer with feeding.
- Protect drug from light.

Anticonvulsants

Clonazepam

Brand Name

Klonopin

Forms

Tablets 0.5 mg, 1 mg, 5 mg (can be made into oral suspension).

Uses

Anticonvulsant. Control of seizures refractory to other anticonvulsants (petit mal, myoclonic, tonic-clonic seizures, and infantile spasms).

Dose

10–30 mcg/kg/day PO q 8–12 hours.
Dose is increased every 3–7 days until seizures are controlled or maximum dose of 200 mcg/kg/day is reached or toxicity occurs.

Pharmacokinetics

Well absorbed from the GI tract. Onset of action is within 20–60 minutes. Steady-state serum level is

reached with 4–12 days. Half-life is 19–60 hours. Largely metabolized in the liver to inactive metabolites. Small amounts are excreted unchanged in the urine. Moderately plasma protein bound.
Therapeutic serum concentration: 20–80 ng/ml.

Cautions

Can cause sedation and drowsiness. May increase the incidence of tonic-clonic seizures in infants with mixed seizure disorders. Can also cause abnormal eye movements, hypotonia, increased salivation, and increased bronchial secretions. Rarely causes diarrhea, constipation, blood dyscrasias (leukopenia, anemia, thrombocytopenia), and transient elevation of liver function tests.

Dependence can occur with long-term use; do not discontinue drug abruptly.

Adaptation to drug, with breakthrough seizures, can occur with long-term use.

Use with caution in infants with liver dysfunction or pulmonary disease.

Drug Interactions

Cimetidine: effects of clonazepam may be increased with excessive sedation.

Nursing Considerations

- Shake suspension well before drawing up dose.
- Administer drug with feeding.
- Observe for seizure activity.
- Assess level of consciousness and tone.
- Monitor pulmonary status. Assess patency of airways; suction prn.

- Monitor liver function and hematologic status.
- Monitor serum drug concentration weekly until control of seizures and steady state reached. Obtain blood just before a dose (trough).
- Refrigerate suspension (stable for 14 days).

Diazepam

Brand Names

Valium, various

Forms

Injection 5 mg/ml (contains propylene glycol and benzyl alcohol).

Uses

Anticonvulsant. Control of seizures refractory to phenobarbital and phenytoin (tonic-clonic seizures and status epilepticus). Short-term use.

Dose

0.2 mg/kg/dose IV. May repeat dose q 2–5 minutes to a maximum of 1 mg/kg.

Pharmacokinetics

Onset of action is within 1–5 minutes. Half-life is 20–50 hours in the term infant, 40–400 hours in the preterm infant. Metabolized in the liver to an active metabolite and excreted by the kidneys. Highly plasma protein bound.

Cautions

Can cause CNS depression, respiratory depression, and hypotension. Concomitant use with phenobarbital can cause hypoventilation or apnea.

Dependence can occur with long-term use. Do not discontinue drug abruptly, may cause seizures. Symptoms of withdrawal may not appear for several days due to drug's long half-life.

Can cause local irritation and phlebitis at injection site.

Use with caution in infants with liver or kidney dysfunction.

Solution Compatibility

Do NOT mix with any IV solutions.

Additive Compatibility

Do NOT mix with other drugs.

Drug Interactions

Cimetidine: effects of diazepam may be increased with excessive sedation.

Nursing Considerations

- Infuse slowly IV push over 3–5 minutes.
- Flush IV with NS before and after administration.
- Observe IV site for extravasation.
- Do NOT administer intraarterially. Can cause arteriospasm and necrosis.
- Observe for seizure activity.
- Assess level of consciousness.
- Monitor respiratory status and BP.
- Monitor liver and kidney function.
- Drug is adsorbed to plastic of IV bags and tubing.
- Protect from light.

Lorazepam

Brand Name

Ativan

Forms

Injection 2 mg/ml (contains propylene glycol and benzyl alcohol).

Uses

Anticonvulsant. Control of seizures refractory to phenobarbital and phenytoin. Short-term use.
Sedation.

Dose

0.05–0.1 mg/kg/dose IV q 4–6 hours based on infant's response.

Pharmacokinetics

Onset of action is within 1–5 minutes. Duration of action is 3–24 hours. Half-life is 10–20 hours. Highly lipid-soluble, enhancing penetration into the CNS. Metabolized in the liver to inactive metabolites and excreted by the kidneys.

Cautions

Can cause CNS and respiratory depression. Concomitant use with phenobarbital can cause hypoventilation or apnea.
   Dependence can occur with long-term use. Do not discontinue drug abruptly, may cause seizures.
   Use with caution in infants with liver dysfunction.

Solution Compatibility

D5W, 0.9% NaCl.

Additive Compatibility

Do NOT mix with other drugs.

Nursing Considerations

- Infuse slowly IV push over 3–5 minutes.
- Dilute drug with an equal volume of compatible diluent (D5W, 0.9% NaCl) just prior to administration.
- Do NOT administer intraarterially. Can cause arteriospasm and necrosis.
- Observe for seizure activity.
- Assess need for sedation:
  – agitation.
  – change in vital signs (increased HR, RR, BP).
  – decreased TcO_2 and/or O_2 saturation, increased $TcCO_2$.
- Assess level of consciousness.
- Monitor respiratory status.
- Monitor liver function.
- Refrigerate drug.
- Protect from light.

Phenobarbital

Brand Names

Various

Forms

Injection 30 mg/ml, 60 mg/ml, 65 mg/ml (contains propylene glycol, benzyl alcohol, and other
preservatives).
Elixir 20 mg/5 ml. Other concentrations are available.

Uses

Anticonvulsant. Control of seizures (tonic-clonic seizures and status epilepticus). Drug of choice for
infants with seizures.
Treatment of significant neonatal drug withdrawal
(SLEEPLESSNESS, progressive irritability, tremoring,
SEIZURES, POOR FEEDING, vomiting, diarrhea, and
WEIGHT LOSS or POOR WEIGHT GAIN or Neonatal
Abstinence Score $\geq$ 8 for 3 consecutive scores or for
an average of 3 consecutive scores). Used in infants
exposed to multiple drugs. Drug of choice for infants
with seizures.

Dose

Anticonvulsant
Loading dose: 10–20 mg/kg IV.
Additional 5 mg/kg doses to a maximum of 40 mg/kg for refractory
seizures.
Initial maintenance dose: 3–5 mg/kg/day IV, PO q 12–
24 hours.
Start maintenance no earlier than 12 hours after
loading dose.
Maintenance dose should be determined by the
infant's serum concentration.

Central Nervous System (CNS) Drugs   **29**

Neonatal Withdrawal

Loading dose: 10–20 mg/kg IV, PO.
                      Additional 10 mg/kg doses to a maximum of 40 mg/kg for control of seizures.

Maintenance: 4–6 mg/kg/day PO q 6–8 hours.
                      Adjust dose for control of withdrawal symptoms.

Irritability and tremors should NOT be the only criteria for initiating drug therapy or adjusting dose.
Maintain effective dose for 3–5 days before reducing dose. Dose is reduced every 1–2 days as tolerated (infant sleeps and feeds well and gains weight). Duration of therapy is usually 10–14 days (longer in infants with seizures due to withdrawal).

Pharmacokinetics

Onset of action is within 1–5 minutes after IV administration. Half-life of 40–200 hours has been reported. Half-life decreases with age. Largely metabolized in the liver to an inactive metabolite; 20–30% is excreted unchanged in the urine. Acid urine may decrease, and alkaline urine increase the excretion of unchanged drug. A maintenance dose of 3 mg/kg/day will produce an initial serum concentration of 20–25 mcg/ml at a steady-state; a dose of 5 mg/kg/day will produce a concentration of 30–35 mcg/ml.
Therapeutic serum concentration: 15–30 mcg/ml.

Cautions

Rapid IV infusion can cause respiratory depression and/or hypotension.

Rash with hypersensitivity.

Sedation and lethargy with drug levels >40 mcg/ml. Coma and respiratory depression with drug levels >60 mcg/ml.

Use with caution in infants with liver or kidney dysfunction.

Solution Compatibility

Dextrose-saline combinations, D5W, D10W, 0.45% NaCl, 0.9% NaCl.

Additive Compatibility

Do NOT mix with other drugs.

Drug Interactions

Aminophylline/Theophylline: effects of aminophylline may be decreased with possible reduced plasma levels.

Dexamethasone: effects of dexamethasone may be decreased.

Propranolol: effects of propranolol may be decreased. The above interactions may occur up to several days after discontinuation of phenobarbital.

Nursing Considerations

- Infuse slowly IV push ≤1 mg/kg/minute.
- Monitor respirations and BP during IV administration.
- Administer PO preparation with feeding.
- Observe for seizure activity.
- Assess level of consciousness and respiratory status.

Central Nervous System (CNS) Drugs   **31**

- Monitor liver and kidney function.
- Monitor serum drug concentration. Obtain blood just prior to a dose (trough).
- Provide parents with written instructions for administering phenobarbital (see Appendix D: Drug Information for Parents).
- Osmolality (elixir 20 mg/5 ml): 11,645 mOsm/kg H_2O (FP).
  (injection 65 mg/ml): 15,570 mOsm/kg H_2O (FP).

For Neonatal Withdrawal

- Onset of withdrawal is shortly after birth to 2 weeks (usually within 72 hours).
- Obtain urine for toxicology on suspected infants.
- Utilize Neonatal Abstinence Score to identify significant withdrawal. Observe infant for SLEEPLESSNESS, excessive or continuous high-pitched crying, hyperactivity, moderate to severe tremoring (especially when undisturbed), hypertonia, SEIZURES, POOR FEEDING, vomiting, diarrhea, WEIGHT LOSS, or POOR WEIGHT GAIN.
- Provide supportive treatment for withdrawal: swaddling, minimal noise and light, waterbed, pacifier, frequent feedings, holding and rocking.
- Monitor caloric intake and daily weights.
- During the initiation and maintenance of drug therapy: monitor HR, rhythm, rate and quality of respirations, color, perfusion, activity, tone, and level of consciousness.
- During reduction of drug therapy: observe for increased signs of withdrawal. Infant should continue to sleep and feed well and gain weight.

Phenytoin

Brand Names

Dilantin, various

Forms

Injection 50 mg/ml (contains propylene glycol, may contain preservatives).
Oral suspension 30 mg/5 ml, 125 mg/5 ml.

Uses

Anticonvulsant. Control of seizures refractory to phenobarbital (tonic-clonic seizures and status epilepticus).

Dose

Loading dose: 10–20 mg/kg IV.
Initial maintenance dose: 4–8 mg/kg/day IV, PO q 12–24 hours.
Start maintenance 12–24 hours after loading dose.
Maintenance dose should be determined by the infant's serum concentration.
Doses to 8 mg/kg or greater q 8–12 hours may be required for older infants.

Pharmacokinetics

Onset of action is within 5–10 minutes after IV administration. Slow and variable absorption from GI tract. Half-life is 8–197 hours, decreasing with age. Rapidly changing and variable rates of elimination in the neonatal period. Largely metabolized in the liver to an inactive metabolite; <10% is excreted unchanged in

the urine. Highly plasma protein bound. Bilirubin will displace drug from protein-binding sites.
Therapeutic serum concentration: 10–20 mcg/ml.

Cautions

Rapid IV infusion can cause bradycardia, arrhythmias, and hypotension.

Hypersensitivity with long-term use (abnormal liver function and blood dyscrasias, i.e., leukopenia, anemia, thrombocytopenia).

Toxic levels can cause vomiting, nystagmus, lethargy, increased seizure activity, cardiac arrhythmias, hypotension, hyperglycemia, and hypoinsulinemia.

Very hyperosmolar; can cause irritation at injection site.

Use with caution in infants with liver dysfunction.

Solution Compatibility

Do NOT mix with any IV solutions.

Additive Compatibility

Do NOT mix with other drugs.

Drug Interactions

Aminophylline/Theophylline: effects of both drugs may be decreased with reduced plasma levels.
Chloramphenicol: effects of phenytoin are increased with possible elevated plasma levels and toxicity. Effects of chloramphenicol may be altered with decreased or increased serum levels.
Cimetidine: effects of phenytoin may be increased with possible elevated plasma levels and toxicity.

Dexamethasone: effects of dexamethasone may be decreased. Effects of phenytoin may be altered; may cause or decrease plasma levels.

Dopamine: action of dopamine may be decreased. Severe hypotension and bradycardia may occur with the administration of phenytoin IV.

Folic Acid: reduced plasma levels and therapeutic effectiveness of phenytoin.

Methadone: effects of methadone may be decreased with possible precipitation of methadone withdrawal. Effect of interaction may occur up to several days after discontinuation of phenytoin.

Rifampin: effects of phenytoin may be decreased with possible reduced plasma levels. Effect of interaction may occur up to several days after discontinuation of phenytoin.

Skeletal muscle relaxants (atracurium, pancuronium, vecuronium): possible resistance to, or reversal of, the neuromuscular blocking effects of nondepolarizing muscle relaxants.

Trimethoprim: effects of phenytoin may be increased with possible elevated plasma levels and toxicity.

Nursing Considerations

- Infuse slowly IV push over 5–10 minutes (≤ 0.5 mg/kg/minute).
- Do not administer IM.
- Monitor HR, rhythm, and BP during IV administration.
- Flush IV with NS before and after administration (contact with any dextrose will cause immediate precipitation).
- Observe IV site for extravasation.

- Oral suspension must be shaken vigorously prior to drawing up dose.
- Administer PO preparation with feeding.
- Observe for seizure activity.
- Monitor level of consciousness.
- Monitor liver function, hematologic status, blood glucose, and serum albumin.
- Monitor serum drug concentration. Obtain blood just before a dose (trough).
- Osmolality (Dilantin suspension 30 mg/5 ml): 2045 mOsm/kg H_2O (FP).
  (Dilantin injection 50 mg/ml): 9740 mOsm/kg H_2O (FP).

Pyridoxine (Vitamin B₆)

Brand Names

Various

Forms

Injection 100 mg/ml (contains benzyl alcohol).
Dilute injectable form for PO use.

Uses

Diagnosis and treatment of pyridoxine-dependent seizures.

Dose

Initial dose: 50–100 mg IV.
Maintenance: 10–100 mg PO QD. Increased dose may be required with intercurrent illness and with growth.

Pharmacokinetics

Seizure usually ceases within 10 minutes (up to 1 hour) after IV administration. Readily absorbed from the GI tract. Metabolized in the liver and excreted by the kidneys.

Cautions

No known side effects with therapeutic doses.

Solution Compatibility

Dextrose-saline combinations, D5W, D10W, 0.9% NaCl.

Additive Incompatibility

Alkaline solutions, iron salts, oxidizing agents.

Nursing Considerations

- Infuse slowly IV push over 2 minutes.
- Ideally, infant should have an EEG in progress during the administration of initial dose.
- Observe infant for 30 minutes after initial dose before administration of anticonvulsants, unless severe seizure activity continues.
- Administer PO preparation with feeding.
- Average onset of pyridoxine-dependent seizures is 4 hours of age (varies from birth to 3 months).
- Protect from light.
- Osmolality (injection 100 mg/ml): 870 mOsm/kg H_2O (FP).

Narcotic Antagonists

Naloxone

Brand Names

Narcan, various

Forms

Injection (neonatal) 0.02 mg/ml.

Uses

Narcotic antagonist. Treatment of narcotic-induced CNS and respiratory depression.

Dose

0.01–0.02 mg/kg/dose (0.5–1 ml/kg of Narcan Neonatal) IV, IM, SQ.
May repeat dose q 3–5 minutes if no response. Subsequent doses should be based on clinical assessment and response of infant.

Pharmacokinetics

Onset of action is within 1–2 minutes after IV administration; 15–40 minutes after IM, SQ administration. Duration of action is short and variable, 1–4 hours. Half-life is 3 hours. Rapidly metabolized in the liver and excreted by the kidneys.

Cautions

Use with caution in infants born to suspected "dependent" mothers. Administration of drug may precipitate withdrawal symptoms in these infants.

Solution Compatibility

D5W, 0.9% NaCl.

Additive Compatibility

Do NOT mix with other drugs.

Nursing Considerations

- Intramuscular and SQ routes are contraindicated in infants with hypotension or shock.
- Observe for CNS and respiratory depression and the need for additional dosing. Half-life of naloxone is shorter than that of most narcotics.
- Observe for acute withdrawal symptoms (jitteriness, hyperactivity, irritability, hypertonicity).
- Protect from light.

Stimulants

Aminophylline (Hydrous and Anhydrous)

Brand Names

Somophyllin, various

Forms

Injection (hydrous) 25 mg/ml (19.7 mg anhydrous theophylline).
Oral solution (anhydrous) 105 mg/5 ml (90 mg anhydrous theophylline).

Uses

Management of apnea of prematurity.
Bronchodilator for infants with BPD.
Facilitate weaning from assisted ventilation.

Dose

Loading dose: 6 mg/kg (5 mg/kg anhydrous theophylline) IV.
Initial maintenance dose: 1.2–3.5 mg/kg/dose IV, PO (1–3 mg/kg anhydrous theophylline) q 8–12 hours. Start maintenance 8–12 hours after loading dose. Maintenance dose should be determined by infant's serum concentration and clinical condition (persistence of apnea vs evidence of toxicity).
Doses to 25 mg/kg/day, q 4–8 hours, may be required for infants > 2–4 months adjusted age.

Pharmacokinetics

Onset of action is within 15 minutes after IV loading dose. Half-life is 12–64 hours (mean 19–32 hours). Metabolized in the liver, in part to caffeine (major metabolite of theophylline in the neonate); > 50% of drug is excreted unchanged in the urine of the preterm infant, decreasing at term. Theophylline clearance increases throughout the first year of life.
Therapeutic serum concentration: Apnea 5–12 mcg/ml (concentrations as low as 3 mcg/ml have been effective). Bronchodilatation 10–20 mcg/ml.

Cautions

Can cause tachycardia (> 180 bpm), irritability, failure to gain weight, vomiting, abdominal distention, GI bleeding, diuresis with dehydration, hyperglycemia, and glycosuria. Jitteriness and hyperreflexia can occur with levels > 20 mcg/ml; cardiac arrhythmias and seizures can occur with levels > 40 mcg/ml.

Theophylline-induced seizures are refractory to anti-convulsants.

Solution Compatibility

Dextrose-saline combinations, D5W, D10W, D20W, 0.45% NaCl, 0.9% NaCl, TPN, fat emulsion 10%.

Additive Compatibility

Calcium gluconate, chloramphenicol, dexamethasone, dopamine, heparin, lidocaine, phenobarbital, potassium chloride, sodium bicarbonate.

Additive Incompatibility

Cefotaxime, cimetidine, clindamycin, dobutamine, epinephrine, hydralazine, isoproterenol, methadone, meperidine, morphine, penicillin G.

Drug Interactions

See "Drug Interactions" for Theophylline.

Nursing Considerations

- Obtain initial serum concentration within 48–72 hours of loading dose. Obtain blood just before a dose (trough).
- Infuse slowly IV over 15–20 minutes.
- Administer PO preparation with feeding to decrease gastric irritation.
- Aminophylline hydrous is 78.9% (± 1.6%) anhydrous theophylline.

- Aminophylline anhydrous is 85.7% (± 1.7%) anhydrous theophylline.
- Dose may need to be adjusted when drug therapy is changed to an anhydrous theophylline preparation.
- Monitor serum drug concentration. Obtain blood just before a dose (trough). Indications for drug monitoring include persistence or recurrence of apnea or evidence of toxicity.
- Monitor for and record apneic episodes (frequency, severity, interventions).
- Observe for signs of toxicity:
  - monitor HR and rhythm.
  - assess activity and tone.
  - observe for gastric signs (gastric residuals, vomiting, abdominal distention, gastric secretions, or stools positive for occult blood).
  - weigh daily.
  - monitor urine output.
  - monitor blood and urine glucose.
- Provide parents with written instructions for administering theophylline (see Appendix D: Drug Information for Parents).

Caffeine Citrate

Brand Names

Various

Forms

Powder (compounding required to make IV and PO preparations).

Caffeine citrate powder contains 50% active caffeine base.

Uses

Management of apnea of prematurity.

Dose

Loading dose: 20 mg/kg IV, PO (10 mg/kg of *active caffeine base*).
Maintenance: 5 mg/kg/day IV, PO (2.5 mg/kg day of *active caffeine base*) QD.
Start maintenance 24 hours after loading dose.
Maintenance dose should be determined by infant's serum concentration and clinical condition (persistence of apnea vs evidence of toxicity).

Pharmacokinetics

Rapidly and well absorbed from the GI tract. Half-life is 37–231 hours (mean > 60 hours). Little to no metabolism. Largely excreted unchanged in the urine of the neonate (to 85%). Caffeine clearance increases between 1 month and 4–6 months of age.
Therapeutic serum concentration: 5–25 mcg/ml (concentrations as low as 3 mcg/ml have been effective).

Cautions

Toxicity with levels > 40–50 mcg/ml. Acute overdose can cause tachycardia, fine tremors, opisthotonus, and seizures.
  Jitteriness with levels > 50 mcg/ml. Tachycardia with levels > 100 mcg/ml.

Solution Compatibility

Dextrose-saline combinations, D5W, D10W, 0.9% NaCl.

Additive Compatibility

Do NOT mix IV preparation with other drugs.

Nursing Considerations

- Obtain initial serum level 24 hours after loading dose. Obtain blood just before a dose (trough).
- Infuse slowly IV over 15–20 minutes.
- Administer PO preparation with feeding.
- Monitor serum drug concentration. Obtain blood just before a dose (trough). Indications for drug monitoring include persistence or recurrence of apnea or evidence of toxicity.
- Monitor for and record apneic episodes (frequency, severity, interventions).
- Observe for signs of toxicity:
  - monitor HR.
  - assess activity and tone.

Doxapram

Brand Name

Dopram

Forms

Injection 20 mg/ml (contains benzyl alcohol).

Uses

Management of apnea of prematurity refractory to therapeutic serum levels of aminophylline, theophylline, or caffeine.

Dose

1–1.5 mg/kg/hour to a maximum of 2.5 mg/kg/hour.
Continuous IV infusion.
When control of apnea is achieved for > 24 hours,
decrease dose as tolerated (0.5 mg/kg/hour has been
effective when used with aminophylline, theophylline,
or caffeine).

Pharmacokinetics

Onset of action is within 20–40 seconds. Duration of
action is < 1 hour, necessitating a continuous IV infusion. Half-life is 5–13 hours. Rapidly metabolized in
the liver and excreted by the kidneys.
Therapeutic serum concentration: < 5 mcg/ml.

Cautions

Toxic levels can cause tachycardia, arrhythmias,
abdominal distention, vomiting, increased gastric
residuals, irritability, jitteriness, seizures, hypertension,
hyperglycemia, and glycosuria.
   Doxapram-induced seizures are responsive to anti-
convulsants.
   Can cause irritation at injection site.
   Use with caution during the first week of life in the
preterm infant because of the risk of an IVH due to
hypertension.

Solution Compatibility

D5W, D10W, 0.9% NaCl.

Additive Compatibility

Do NOT mix with other drugs.

Drug Interactions

Concomitant use with vasopressors may cause synergistic pressor effect.

Nursing Considerations

- Maintain a continuous IV infusion.
- Observe IV site for extravasation.
- Monitor for and record apneic episodes (frequency, severity, interventions).
- Observe for signs of toxicity:
  - monitor HR and BP.
  - assess activity and tone (abnormal jerky limb movements precede seizures).
  - observe for gastric signs (gastric residuals, vomiting, abdominal distention).
  - monitor blood and urine glucose.

Theophylline (Anhydrous)

Brand Names

Various

Forms

Syrups, elixirs, and liquids 50 mg/ml, 80 mg/15 ml, 150 mg/5 ml (may contain alcohol and preservatives).

Uses

Management of apnea of prematurity.
Bronchodilator for infants with BPD.
Facilitate weaning from assisted ventilation.

Dose

Loading dose: 5 mg/kg PO.
Initial maintenance dose: 1–3 mg/kg/dose PO
q 8–12 hours.
Start maintenance 8–12 hours after loading dose.
Maintenance dose should be determined by infant's
serum concentration and clinical condition (persistence of apnea vs evidence of toxicity).
Doses to 25 mg/kg/day, q 4–8 hours, may be required
for infants > 2–4 months adjusted age.

Pharmacokinetics

Variable rate of absorption from the GI tract after PO
administration, with 80–100% bioavailability. Half-life is
12–64 hours (mean 19–32 hours). Metabolized in the
liver, in part to caffeine (major metabolite of theophylline in the neonate); > 50% of drug is excreted
unchanged in the urine of the preterm infant,
decreasing at term. Theophylline clearance increases
throughout the first year of life.
Therapeutic serum concentration: Apnea 5–12 mcg/ml
(concentrations as
low as 3 mcg/ml
have been effec-
tive).
Bronchodilatation
10–20 mcg/ml.

Cautions

Can cause tachycardia (> 180 bpm), irritability, failure
to gain weight, vomiting, abdominal distention, GI
bleeding, diuresis with dehydration, hyperglycemia,

and glycosuria. Jitteriness and hyperreflexia can occur with levels > 20 mcg/ml; cardiac arrhythmias and seizures can occur with levels > 40 mcg/ml.

Theophylline-induced seizures are refractory to anti-convulsants.

Drug Interactions

Cimetidine: effect of theophylline may be increased with possible elevated plasma levels and toxicity.
Erythromycin: effects of theophylline may be increased with possible elevated plasma levels and toxicity. Effectiveness of erythromycin may also be decreased.
Halothane: toxicity (cardiac arrhythmias) of theophylline may be increased (theophylline dose dependent).
Phenobarbital: effects of theophylline may be decreased with possible reduced plasma levels. Effect of interaction may occur up to several days after the discontinuation of phenobarbital.
Phenytoin: effects of both drugs may be reduced with reduced plasma levels of both drugs.
Propranolol: theophylline level may be reduced.
Rifampin: effects of theophylline may be decreased with reduced plasma levels. Effects of interaction may occur up to several days after discontinuation of rifampin.
Skeletal muscle relaxants (atracurium, pancuronium, vecuronium): possible resistance to, or reversal of, neuromuscular blocking effects of nondepolarizing muscle relaxants (theophylline dose dependent).

Nursing Considerations

- Obtain initial serum concentration within 48–72 hours of loading dose. Obtain blood just before a dose (trough).
- Administer with feeding to decrease gastric irritation.
- Dose may need to be adjusted when drug therapy is changed to an aminophylline hydrous or anhydrous preparation (see "Aminophylline").
- Monitor serum drug concentration. Obtain blood just before a dose (trough). Indications for drug monitoring include persistence or recurrence of apnea or evidence of toxicity.
- Monitor for and record apneic episodes (frequency, severity, interventions).
- Observe for signs of toxicity:
  - monitor HR and rhythm.
  - assess activity and tone.
  - observe for gastric signs (gastric residuals, vomiting, abdominal distention, gastric secretions, or stools positive for occult blood).
  - weigh daily.
  - monitor urine output.
  - monitor blood and urine glucose.
- Provide parents with written instructions for administering theophylline (see Appendix D: Drug Information for Parents).
- Osmolality (Theostat80 syrup 80 mg/15 ml): 4985 mOsm/kg H_2O (FP).

Chapter 3

Cardiovascular (CV) Drugs

Antiarrhythmics

Lidocaine

Brand Names

Xylocaine, various

Forms

Injection 100 mg/5 ml (2% solution).

Uses

Antiarrhythmic. Drug of choice for acute treatment of ventricular arrhythmias (ventricular tachycardia and premature ventricular contractions).
Also effective with digoxin-induced atrial and ventricular arrhythmias. Short-term use.
Enhances electrical defibrillation in the presence of ventricular fibrillation.

Dose

Initial dose: 1 mg/kg/dose IV. May repeat in 10 minutes prn. Maximum initial dose is 5 mg/kg.

Maintenance: 10–50 mcg/kg/minute. Continuous IV infusion.

Decreases myocardial irritability and abolishes ventricular reentry.

ECG effects include: decreased PR ($\pm$) and QT ($\pm$) intervals.

Hemodynamic effects include: decreased BP ($\pm$) and cardiac output ($\pm$).

Pharmacokinetics

Onset of action is 1–5 minutes after IV administration. Poorly absorbed from the GI tract; not administered PO. Half-life is 15–30 minutes (up to 3 hours in the preterm infant). Metabolized in the liver to active metabolites (monoethylglycinexylidide [MEGX] and glycinexylidide [GX]) with antiarrhythmic activity. Both metabolites can contribute to CNS toxicity. Twenty to thirty percent of drug is excreted unchanged in urine of the neonate. Moderately plasma protein bound. Therapeutic serum concentration: 2–6 mcg/ml.

Cautions

Toxicity with levels > 9 mcg/ml. Levels > 6 mcg/ml can cause drowsiness or agitation, tremors, and vomiting. Levels > 9 mcg/ml can cause bradycardia, asystole, hypotension, arrhythmias, seizures, and respiratory depression or apnea.

Contraindicated in infants with heart failure or heart block.

Use with caution in infants with liver or kidney dysfunction.

Solution Compatibility

D5W, 0.45% NaCl, 0.9% NaCl.

Additive Compatibility

Aminophylline, calcium, carbenicillin, chloramphenicol, cimetidine, dexamethasone, digoxin, dobutamine,
dopamine, heparin, hydrocortisone, methicillin, metoclopramide, penicillin G, procainamide, sodium
bicarbonate.

Additive Incompatibility

Ampicillin.

Drug Interactions

Cimetidine: effects of lidocaine may be increased with
possible elevated plasma levels of lidocaine and toxicity.
Propranolol: see "*Cimetidine.*"
Succinylcholine: neuromuscular blocking effects of
succinylcholine may be increased. Prolonged respiratory depression with extended periods of apnea may
occur (lidocaine dose dependent).

Nursing Considerations

- Infuse slowly IV push over 5–10 minutes.
- Stop or decrease IV infusion if undesirable effects
  occur.
- Use controlled infusion device for continuous IV
  infusion.
- Quick solution dilution: # **mg** of lidocaine to add to
  100 ml IV solution = weight
  (kg) × # mcg/kg/minute ×
  6, at infusion rate of 1 ml/
  hour.

  If volume of drug to be added to 100 ml IV solution

is >10 ml (>10% of total volume), adjust IV solution volume so total volume equals 100 ml.
- Monitor ECG, HR, BP, and RR continuously. Obtain baseline and intermittent lead 2 rhythm strip. Measure PR and QT intervals.
- Assess level of consciousness.
- Observe for seizure activity.
- Monitor liver and kidney function with long-term use.
- Do not use if discolored or contains precipitate.

Phenytoin

Brand Names

Dilantin, various

Forms

Injection 50 mg/ml (contains propylene glycol, may contain preservatives).
Oral suspension 30 mg/5 ml, 125 mg/5 ml.

Uses

Antiarrhythmic. Drug of choice for treatment of digoxin-induced atrial, ventricular, and junctional arrhythmias. Treatment of ventricular arrhythmias, especially ventricular tachycardia.

Dose

Initial dose: 2–5 mg/kg/dose IV. May repeat q 10 minutes prn. Maximum initial dose is 20 mg/kg.
Maintenance: 2–8 mg/kg/day PO q 8–12 hours.
    Decreases AV conduction and suppresses ectopic beats.

Cardiovascular (CV) Drugs   **53**

ECG effects include: decreased PR (±) and QT intervals.

Hemodynamic effects include: decreased BP (±) and cardiac output (±).

Pharmacokinetics

Onset of action is within 5–10 minutes after IV administration. Slow and variable absorption from the GI tract. Half-life is 8–197 hours, decreasing with age. Rapidly changing and variable rates of elimination in the neonatal period. Largely metabolized in the liver to an inactive metabolite; < 10% is excreted unchanged in the urine. Highly plasma protein bound.
Therapeutic serum concentration (for antiarrhythmic activity): 5–18 mcg/ml.

Cautions

Rapid IV infusion can cause bradycardia, arrhythmias, and hypotension. Toxicity can cause vomiting, nystagmus, lethargy, tremors, arrhythmias, hypotension, hyperglycemia, and hypoinsulinemia.

Hypersensitivity with long-term use (abnormal liver function and blood dyscrasias, i.e., leukopenia, anemia, thrombocytopenia).

Very hyperosmolar; can cause irritation at injection site.

Contraindicated in infants with complete heart block.

Use with caution in infants with liver dysfunction.

Solution Compatibility

Do NOT mix with any IV solution.

Additive Compatibility

Do NOT mix with other drugs.

Drug Interactions

See "Drug Interactions" of phenytoin (anticonvulsant use).

Nursing Considerations

- Infuse slowly IV push over 5–10 minutes (< 0.5 mg/kg/minute).
- Do not administer IM.
- Monitor ECG, HR, and BP, especially during IV administration. Obtain baseline and intermittent lead 2 rhythm strip. Measure PR and QT intervals.
- Flush IV with NS before and after administration (contact with any dextrose will cause immediate precipitation).
- Observe IV site for extravasation.
- Oral suspension must be shaken vigorously prior to drawing up dose.
- Administer PO preparation with feeding.
- Assess level of consciousness.
- Monitor liver function, hematologic status, blood glucose, and serum albumin.
- Monitor serum drug concentration. Obtain blood just before a dose (trough).
- Osmolality (Dilantin suspension 30 mg/5 ml): 2045 mOsm/kg H_2O (FP).
  (Dilantin injection 50 mg/ml): 9740 mOsm/kg H_2O (FP).

Procainamide

Brand Names

Pronestyl, various

Forms

Injection 100 mg/ml (may contain preservatives). Capsules 250 mg, 500 mg (can be made into oral suspension).

Uses

Antiarrhythmic. Treatment of supraventricular arrhythmias (paroxysmal atrial tachycardia and atrial fibrillation) and ventricular tachycardia. Short-term use.

Dose

Initial dose: 1 mg/kg/dose IV q 5 minutes to maximum of 10–15 mg/kg.

Maintenance: 20–50 mcg/kg/minute. Continuous IV infusion.
15–50 mg/kg/day PO q 4–6 hours.

Decreases myocardial excitability and conduction velocity. May depress myocardial contractility.

ECG effects include: increased PR (±) and QT intervals and QRS duration.

Hemodynamic effects include: decreased BP and cardiac output.

Pharmacokinetics

Onset of action is 1–5 minutes after IV administration; within 1 hour after PO administration. Rapidly and completely absorbed from the GI tract (75–90%). Half-life is 2–4 hours. Fifty to sixty percent is excreted unchanged in the urine with metabolites; 40% is metabolized in the liver, in part, to an active metabolite (N-acetylprocainamide [NAPA]) with antiarrhythmic activity like parent drug. Half-life of metabolite is ~ 6 hours.

Therapeutic serum concentration: 3–10 mcg/ml (NAPA serum level: 5–30 mcg/ml).

Cautions

Toxicity with levels > 12 mcg/ml. Levels > 12 mcg/ml can cause poor feeding, vomiting, diarrhea, weakness, and mild hypotension. Levels > 16 mcg/ml can cause hypotension, bradycardia, AV conduction disturbances, ventricular arrhythmias, and asystole. Toxicity can also cause fever, rashes, and agranulocytosis (rare, but potentially fatal).

Long-term use (> 1 year) causing drug-induced systemic lupus erythematosus (rash, fever, pericarditis, pleuritis) has been reported in adults.

Rapid IV infusion can cause decreased myocardial contractility and hypotension.

Contraindicated in infants with 2° or 3° heart block.

Use with caution in infants with heart failure or kidney or liver dysfunction.

Solution Compatibility

D5W, 0.9% NaCl.

Additive Compatibility

Dobutamine, lidocaine.

Cardiovascular (CV) Drugs

Drug Interactions

Cimetidine: pharmacologic effects of procainamide may be increased with possible elevated procainamide and NAPA plasma levels with toxicity.

Nursing Considerations

- Infuse slowly IV push over 5 minutes.
- Stop or decrease infusion rate if undesirable effects occur.
- Use controlled infusion device for continuous IV infusion.
- Quick solution dilution: **# mg** of procainamide to add to 100 ml IV solution = weight (kg) × # mcg/kg/minute × 6, at infusion rate of 1 ml/hour.

  If volume of drug to be added to 100 ml IV solution is > 10 ml (> 10% of total volume), adjust IV solution volume so total volume equals 100 ml.
- Monitor HR, rhythm, and BP continuously during IV infusion. Obtain baseline and intermittent lead 2 rhythm strip. Measure PR and QT intervals and QRS duration.
- Administer PO preparation with feeding.
- Monitor serum drug and metabolite concentrations with IV or long-term use.
- Monitor WBC and differential.
- Observe for signs of infection (feeding intolerance, hypothermia or hyperthermia, lethargy, irritability, respiratory distress).
- Monitor liver and kidney function with long-term use.
- Stable in solution for 24 hours.
- Do not use if discolored or contains precipitate.

Propranolol

Brand Names

Inderal, various

Forms

Injection 1 mg/ml.
Oral solution 20 mg/5 ml, 40 mg/5 ml, 80 mg/ml (may contain parabens).
Other extemporaneously prepared forms are available.

Uses

Antiarrhythmic and β-blocking agent. Treatment of supraventricular tachycardia (especially paroxysmal atrial tachycardia) and ventricular arrhythmias; digoxin-induced atrial and ventricular arrhythmias. Often used with digoxin for treatment of supraventricular tachycardia.
Prevention of hypoxemic "spells" in infants with tetralogy of Fallot.

Dose

Initial dose:	0.01–0.1 mg/kg/dose IV. May repeat in 15 minutes prn. Maximum initial dose is 1 mg.
Maintenance:	1–8 mg/kg/day PO q 6–8 hours.
Hypoxemic "spells" Initial dose:	0.15–0.25 mg/kg/dose IV. May repeat in 15 minutes × 1 dose.
Maintenance:	1–2 mg/kg/dose PO q 6 hours.

Decreases myocardial excitability and conduction and myocardial contractility.

ECG effects include: increased PR (±) and decreased QT (±) intervals.

Hemodynamic effects include: decreased HR, BP (±), and cardiac output.

Pharmacokinetics

Onset of action is within 2–5 minutes after IV administration; within 30–60 minutes after PO administration. Rapid and variable absorption from the GI tract (∼ 30% of drug bioavailable). Half-life is 3–6 hours. Metabolized in the liver, in part, to an active metabolite (4-hydroxypropranolol) with antiarrhythmic activity like parent drug. Half-life of metabolite is 5–7.5 hours. Five percent of drug is excreted unchanged in the urine. Highly plasma protein bound.
Therapeutic serum concentration: 20–100 ng/ml.

Cautions

Toxicity can cause hypotension, bradycardia, asystole, AV conduction disturbances, bronchospasm, possible respiratory depression, acute heart failure, seizures, hypoglycemia, vomiting, diarrhea or constipation, decreased platelet aggregation, and agranulocytosis (rare).

Contraindicated in infants with heart failure or heart block.

Use with caution in infants with kidney or liver dysfunction or obstructive lung disease.

Solution Compatibility

D5W, 0.9% NaCl.

Additive Compatibility

Do NOT mix with other drugs.

Drug Interactions

Aminophylline/theophylline: bronchodilating effect of
theophylline may be decreased. Theophylline plasma
levels may also be reduced.
Cimetidine: effects of propranolol may be increased.
Decreased heart rate, sinus bradycardia, and hypotension may occur.
Epinephrine: effects such as increased systolic and
diastolic blood pressure, marked decrease in heart
rate, and epinephrine resistance may occur.
Hydralazine: effects of both drugs may be increased.
Indomethacin: antihypertensive effectiveness of propranolol may be decreased.
Lidocaine: effects of lidocaine may be increased with
possible elevated plasma levels and toxicity.
Phenobarbital: effects of propranolol may be
decreased. Effect of interaction may occur up to several days after discontinuation of phenobarbital.
Rifampin: effects of propranolol may be decreased.
Effect of interaction may occur up to several days
after discontinuation of rifampin.

Nursing Considerations

- Infuse slowly IV push over 10 minutes.
- Monitor HR, rhythm, and BP. Obtain baseline and

intermittent lead 2 rhythm strip. Measure PR and QT intervals.

- Monitor respiratory status (rate and quality of respirations).
- Administer PO preparation with feedings or immediately after.
- Observe for signs of heart failure: respiratory distress (tachypnea, retractions, wheezing, grunting, flaring), tachycardia, gallop rhythm, peripheral cyanosis, metabolic acidosis, liver enlargement, sweating, lethargy or irritability, poor feeding, and failure to thrive.
- Monitor WBC and differential, platelet count, and blood glucose.
- Observe for signs of infection (feeding intolerance, hypothermia or hyperthermia, lethargy, irritability, respiratory distress).
- Monitor liver and kidney function.

Quinidine Sulfate

Brand Names

Various

Forms

Tablets 200 mg, 300 mg (can be made into oral suspension).

Uses

Antiarrhythmic. Treatment of supraventricular and ventricular arrhythmias. In the treatment of supraventricular tachycardia, quinidine is usually used with digoxin and NOT alone.

Dose

15–60 mg/kg/day PO q 6–8 hours.
Decrease dose if > 50% increase in QRS duration.

Decreases myocardial excitability and conduction velocity. May depress myocardial contractility.

ECG effects include: increased PR ($\pm$) and QT intervals and QRS duration.

Hemodynamic effects include: decreased BP and cardiac output.

Pharmacokinetics

Rapidly and well absorbed from the GI tract (> 90%) with only ~ 30% of drug reaching the circulation due to metabolism on first pass through the liver. Half-life is 4–5 hours. Metabolized in the liver to three active metabolites; 10–30% of drug is excreted unchanged in the urine with metabolites.
Therapeutic serum concentration: 2–6 mcg/ml.

Cautions

An idiosyncratic reaction can occur with first time use characterized by ventricular arrhythmias and syncope.

Toxicity with levels > 9 mcg/ml. Can cause sudden death, bradycardia, asystole, hypotension, arrhythmias, vomiting, diarrhea, poor feeding, abdominal pain, hypersensitivity (rash, fever), blood dyscrasias (thrombocytopenia, hemolytic anemia, agranulocytosis), and cinchonism (auditory and visual impairment, flushing, abdominal pain, vomiting, tremors, respiratory difficulty).

Most common side effects are vomiting and diarrhea which often require discontinuation of drug.

Cardiovascular (CV) Drugs   **63**

Intravenous administration can cause bradycardia and severe hypotension.

Contraindicated in infants with heart failure, heart block, or digoxin toxicity.

Use with caution in infants with liver or kidney dysfunction.

Drug Interactions

Cimetidine: effects of quinidine may be increased with elevated quinidine plasma levels and toxicity.

Digoxin: toxic effects of digoxin may be increased due to increased serum digoxin levels, while inotropic action may be decreased.

Phenobarbital: effects of quinidine may be decreased. Effects of interaction may occur up to several days after discontinuation of phenobarbital.

Phenytoin: effects of quinidine may be decreased. Effects of interaction may occur up to several days after discontinuation of phenytoin.

Rifampin: effects of quinidine may be decreased. Effects of interaction may occur up to several days after discontinuation of rifampin.

Skeletal muscle relaxants (atracurium, pancuronium, vecuronium): neuromuscular blocking effects of nondepolarizing muscle relaxants may be increased. Prolonged respiratory depression with extended periods of apnea may occur.

Succinylcholine: neuromuscular blocking effects of succinylcholine may be increased. Prolonged respiratory depression with extended periods of apnea may occur.

Nursing Considerations

- Do NOT administer IV.
- Monitor ECG, HR, and BP. Obtain baseline and intermittent lead 2 rhythm strip. Measure PR and QT intervals and QRS duration.
- Administer PO preparation with feeding to decrease gastric irritation.
- Observe for vomiting and diarrhea.
- Monitor CBC with differential and platelet count.
- Monitor liver and kidney function.
- Monitor serum drug concentration.

Antihypertensive Agents

Captopril

Brand Name

Capoten

Forms

Tablets 12.5 mg and 25 mg scored (crush and mix with water for PO administration).

Uses

Antihypertensive. Treatment of moderate to severe hypertension refractory to hydralazine and/or diuretics, especially hypertension associated with renovascular abnormalities and hyperreninemia.
Vasodilator (arteriolar/venous). Treatment of refractory CHF (reduces afterload and increases cardiac

output). Used in combination with a cardiac glycoside
and diuretic.

Dose

0.1–1 mg/kg/dose PO q 6–12 hours as needed for
control of BP.
Start with low dose (0.1 mg/kg) and increase gradually for control of BP.

Pharmacokinetics

Approximately 75% of dose is absorbed, rapidly
entering the circulation. Onset of action is within 15
minutes after a single dose. Peak effect occurs
between 30–90 minutes. Duration of action is between
2–6 hours, increasing with additional doses. Partially
metabolized in the liver and excreted in the urine,
40% unchanged and the remainder as metabolites.
Clearance is decreased in infants with kidney dysfunction. Moderately plasma protein bound.

Cautions

Can cause hypotension (especially in volume
depleted infants after the initial dose), rash, fever,
vomiting, constipation, hyperkalemia, proteinuria, and
rarely, neutropenia and agranulocytosis.
  Use with caution in infants with immature or
impaired kidney function and in infants receiving
potassium supplements and/or potassium-sparing
diuretics.
  Contraindicated in infants with bilateral renal artery
thrombosis.

Drug Interactions

Food: antihypertensive effectiveness of captopril may be decreased by food.

Indomethacin: antihypertensive effectiveness of captopril may be decreased or completely abolished, particularly in low-renin hypertension.

Potassium preparations: hyperkalemia may occur with possible cardiac arrhythmias or arrest.

Spironolactone: see "*Potassium preparations.*"

Nursing Considerations

- Crush tablet and mix in water just prior to administration. Draw up desired dose in syringe and discard remaining solution.
  NOTE: Undissolved residue is excipients, not the active drug.
- Administer 1 hour before feeding (food in the GI tract may reduce absorption by 30%).
- Monitor BP prior to administration and at intervals between 15 and 90 minutes after administration, particularly with the initial dose.
- Have volume expansion (blood, plasma, or other colloid) immediately available with administration of initial dose.
- Monitor serum potassium.
- Monitor kidney function.
- Monitor CBC.
- Establish BP limits for each infant for dose administration (i.e., "Hold dose if systolic BP < 80 mm Hg or mean BP < 60 mm Hg").

Hydralazine

Brand Name

Apresoline

Forms

Injection 20 mg/ml (contains preservatives).
Tablets 10 mg, 25 mg (can be made into oral suspension).

Uses

Antihypertensive. Drug of choice for the treatment of mild to moderate hypertension in the neonate and infant.
Vasodilator (arteriolar). Short-term treatment of refractory CHF (reduces afterload and increases cardiac output), used in combination with a cardiac glycoside, diuretic, and/or other vasodilator.

Dose

Hypertension.   0.1–0.5 mg/kg/dose IV, PO q 3–6 hours for BP control. Increase gradually to a maximum dose of 2 mg/kg q 6 hours.
When route changed from IV to PO, an increase of at least 2× the effective IV dose may be necessary.
Vasodilation.   0.1–0.5 mg/kg/dose IV q 6 hours.
Maximum dose: 2 mg/kg q 6 hours.

Pharmacokinetics

Onset of action is within 10–30 minutes after IV administration with peak effect at 30 minutes and duration of action between 2 and 4 hours. Onset of action is within 30–60 minutes after PO administration; duration of action is up to 8 hours. Half-life is 2–4 hours, up to 8 hours. Rapidly absorbed from the GI tract after PO administration and extensively metabolized in the GI mucosa and the liver to inactive metabolites with reduced systemic bioavailability. Metabolites are excreted in the urine with small amounts of unchanged drug. Highly plasma protein bound.

Cautions

Can cause tachycardia, hypotension, vomiting, diarrhea, GI irritation and hemorrhage, sodium and water retention and edema (without concomitant diuretic therapy), nasal congestion, lacrimation, flushing, and rarely, skin rash, fever, anemia, leukopenia, and agranulocytosis. A lupus-like syndrome has been reported in adults.

Use with caution in infants with severe liver, kidney, or heart disease.

Solution Compatibility

Dextrose-saline combinations, D5W, D10W, 0.45% NaCl, 0.9% NaCl.

Additive Compatibility

Do NOT mix with other drugs.

Drug Interactions

Propranolol: effects of both drugs may be increased.

Nursing Considerations

- Infuse slowly IV push over 3 minutes.
- Administer PO preparation with feeding.

Cardiovascular (CV) Drugs　　　　　　　　**69**

- Monitor BP prior to administration of dose and 30–60 minutes after IV route and 1–2 hours after PO route.
- Monitor HR and temperature.
- Monitor daily weights and urine output.
- Check stools and gastric residuals for occult blood.
- Monitor CBC with long-term use.
- Establish BP limits for each infant for dose administration (i.e., "Hold dose if systolic BP < 80 mm Hg or mean BP < 60 mm Hg").

Nitroprusside

Brand Name

Nipride

Forms

Injection 50 mg (powder for reconstitution).

Uses

Antihypertensive. Drug of choice for treatment of hypertensive crisis.
Vasodilator (arteriolar/venous). Short-term use for treatment of refractory CHF (reduces afterload and increases cardiac output).

Dose

0.5–10 mcg/kg/minute. Continuous IV infusion.
Start with low dose (0.5–1 mcg/kg/minute) and titrate to desired effect.
Maximum dose for prolonged use (> 48 hours): 2 mcg/kg/minute.

Do NOT infuse at a rate of 10 mcg/kg/minute for
> 10 minutes.
Decrease dose 15–25%, as tolerated, q 6–12 hours
after 12–24 hours of BP stability.

Pharmacokinetics

Onset of action is within 1–2 minutes. Duration of
action is only minutes, necessitating a continuous
infusion. Rapidly metabolized in various tissues and
the liver and is excreted entirely as metabolites in the
urine. Principal metabolite is thiocyanate with a half-
life of 4–7 days with normal kidney function.

Cautions

Can cause severe hypotension, tachycardia, and
muscle twitching. Can worsen intrapulmonary
shunting. Accumulation of cyanide (RBC levels > 50–
100 nmol/ml) and thiocyanate (serum levels > 5–10
mg/dl) can occur in infants with severe liver or kidney
dysfunction or with prolonged use (> 72 hours),
causing toxicity with metabolic acidosis, increased
venous pO_2, respiratory distress, and seizures.
 Can cause tissue sloughing and necrosis with
extravasation.
 Use with caution in infants with liver or kidney dysfunction.

Solution Compatibility

D5W.

Additive Compatibility

Do NOT mix with other drugs.

Nursing Considerations

- Have volume expansion (plasma, blood, or other colloid) immediately available when infusion is initiated.
- Monitor intraarterial BP CONTINUOUSLY.
- Quick solution dilution: # **mg** of nitroprusside to add to 100 ml IV solution = wt (kg) × # mcg/kg/minute × 6, at infusion rate of 1 ml/ hour.
  If volume of drug to be added to 100 ml IV solution is > 10 ml (> 10% of total volume), adjust IV solution volume so total volume equals 100 ml.
- Stop or decrease infusion rate if undesired effects occur.
- Double-check dose and rate of infusion.
- Maintain continuous IV infusion. Use controlled infusion device for administration.
- Do NOT bolus or piggyback other drugs via nitroprusside infusion.
- Use umbilical vein or large peripheral vein for administration.
- Monitor HR.
- Monitor acid-base balance with blood gases (metabolic acidosis is the earliest, most reliable sign of toxicity) and venous pO_2.
- Monitor kidney and liver function.
- Monitor serum thiocyanate and RBC cyanide levels daily with prolonged use (> 48 hours) and in infants with liver or kidney dysfunction.
- Protect ENTIRE infusion from light with aluminum foil or other opaque material.

- Stable for 24 hours after dilution in a compatible IV solution, with proper protection from light.
- Discard unused portions of reconstituted vial. Use freshly prepared solutions of reconstituted drug.
- Do not use if highly discolored (normally has brownish tint) or contains particulate matter.

Tolazoline

Brand Name

Priscoline

Forms

Injection 25 mg/ml.

Uses

Vasodilator (arteriolar/venous). Management of persistent pulmonary hypertension in the neonate (PPHN) refractory to maximal oxygen and ventilator support (decreases pulmonary artery pressure). Used in conjunction with dopamine.

Dose

Initial dose: 1–2 mg/kg IV bolus over 10 minutes.
A response, if it occurs, should be observed within 30 minutes of initial dose.
Correct acidosis and hypovolemia prior to administration.
Maintenance: 1–2 mg/kg/hour. Continuous IV infusion.
Doses > 5 mg/kg/hour are not likely to increase efficacy.

Cardiovascular (CV) Drugs   73

Start continuous infusion only if positive response (increased pO_2) is observed after initial dose.

Pharmacokinetics

Onset of action is within minutes. Duration of action is between 3–10 hours. Rapidly excreted, largely unchanged, in the urine. Accumulation of drug may occur in infants with kidney dysfunction. Stimulates histamine release.

Cautions

Side effects by body systems include:

CV: hypotension, tachycardia, flushing.

Respiratory: pulmonary hemorrhage, increased salivary and respiratory secretions.

GI: increased gastric secretions, gastric bleeding and/or perforation, vomiting, diarrhea, abdominal distention.

Renal: oliguria, hematuria, edema.

Metabolic: hyponatremia.

Hematologic: thrombocytopenia, agranulocytosis.

Use with caution in infants with kidney dysfunction. Contraindicated in infants with kidney failure, active bleeding, hypotension, or shock.

Solution Compatibility

D5W, D10W, 0.45% NaCl, 0.9% NaCl.

Additive Compatibility

Do NOT mix with other drugs.

Drug Interactions

Epinephrine: large doses of tolazoline administered concurrently with epinephrine may cause a paradoxical fall in BP followed by an exaggerated rebound increase in BP.

Nursing Considerations

- Have volume expansion (plasma, blood, or other colloid) and vasopressor (dopamine) immediately available with administration of initial dose.
- Infuse initial dose slowly over 10 minutes.
- Monitor intraarterial BP CONTINUOUSLY.
- Quick solution dilution: **# mg** of tolazoline to add to 100 ml IV solution = wt (kg) × # mg/kg/hour × 100, at infusion rate of 1 ml/hour.

If volume of drug to be added to 100 ml IV solution is > 10 ml (> 10% of total volume), adjust IV solution volume so total volume equals 100 ml.

- Stop or decrease infusion rate if undesired effects occur.
- Double-check dose and rate of infusion.
- Use controlled infusion device for administration.
- Do NOT bolus or piggyback other drugs via tolazoline infusion.
- Use pulmonary artery or vein that drains into the superior vena cava (scalp or upper extremity vein) for administration.
- Monitor HR.
- Monitor oxygenation, ventilation, and acid-base balance (arterial blood gases, TcO_2, $TcCO_2$, O_2 saturation).
- Check stools and gastric secretions for occult blood.
- Monitor kidney function and urine output.
- Consider prophylactic use of an antacid to prevent

gastric irritation (cimetidine may antagonize tolazo-
line-induced vasodilation).
- Monitor CBC and platelet count.
- Stable for 24 hours after dilution in a compatible IV
solution.

Sympathomimetics

Dobutamine

Brand Name

Dobutrex

Forms

Injection 12.5 mg/ml in 20 ml vials.

Uses

Improvement of cardiac output and blood pressure in
cardiogenic and hypovolemic shock states, refractory
to dopamine. May be used in combination with low to
moderate doses of dopamine (to optimize cardiac
output without increasing peripheral vascular resistance).

Dose

2–10 mcg/kg/minute. Continuous IV infusion.
Start with low dose (2–5 mcg/kg/minute) and titrate to
desired effect.
Correct hypovolemia prior to administration.
    Increases myocardial contractility, blood pressure,
± heart rate, O_2 delivery and consumption. Peripheral
vasoconstriction at low doses; vasodilation at high
doses.

Pharmacokinetics

Onset of action is within 1–2 minutes. Duration of action is 10 minutes, necessitating a continuous IV infusion. Half-life is 2 minutes. Rapidly metabolized in the liver.

Cautions

Can cause tachycardia, arrhythmias (less than dopamine and isoproterenol), increased or decreased blood pressure, and cutaneous vasodilation. Unlike dopamine, dobutamine does not cause renal artery dilation.

Use with caution in infants with liver dysfunction.

Solution Compatibility

D5W, D10W, 0.45% NaCl, 0.9% NaCl.

Additive Compatibility

Dopamine, epinephrine, heparin, isoproterenol, lidocaine, procainamide.

Additive Incompatibility

Aminophylline, calcium gluconate, magnesium sulfate.

Nursing Considerations

• Quick solution dilution: **# mg** of dobutamine to add to 100 ml IV solution = weight (kg) × # mcg/kg/minute × 6, at infusion rate of 1 ml/hour.

If volume of drug to be added to 100 ml IV solution

is > 10 ml (> 10% of total volume), adjust IV solution volume so total volume equals 100 ml.

- Stop or decrease infusion rate if undesired effects occur.
- Double-check dose and rate of infusion.
- Maintain continuous IV infusion. Use controlled infusion device for administration.
- Use large vein for administration.
- Monitor HR, rhythm, and arterial BP continuously.
- Assess capillary refill.
- Monitor for adequate oxygenation, ventilation, and acid-base balance: (blood gases, TcO_2, $TcCO_2$, O_2 saturation).
- Caution when changing solution daily (avoid bolus or prolonged interruption of drug infusion). Monitor closely for changes in BP.
- Do NOT BOLUS other drugs via dobutamine infusion.
- Stable for 24 hours after dilution in a compatible IV solution.

Dopamine

Brand Names

Intropin, various

Forms

Injection 200 mg/5 ml, 400 mg/5 ml, 800 mg/5 ml.

Uses

Improvement of cardiac output, blood pressure, and

kidney perfusion in cardiogenic and hypovolemic shock states.

Dose

2–20 mcg/kg/minute. Continuous IV infusion.
Start with low dose (2–5 mcg/kg/minute) and titrate to desired effect.
Correct hypovolemia prior to administration.

2–5 mcg/kg/minute:	Increases urine output and sodium excretion. Decreases peripheral vascular resistance.
5–10 mcg/kg/minute:	Increases myocardial contractility, ± heart rate, and possibly blood pressure (mainly systolic).
10–20 mcg/kg/minute:	Increases myocardial contractility, blood pressure (mainly systolic), heart rate, and peripheral and possibly pulmonary vascular resistance. Causes renal vasoconstriction.

Pharmacokinetics

Onset of action is within 2–4 minutes. Duration of action is 10 minutes, necessitating a continuous IV infusion. Half-life is 2 minutes. Rapidly metabolized in the liver, kidneys, and plasma. Small amounts of the drug are converted to epinephrine and norepinephrine.

Cautions

Can cause tachycardia, arrhythmias (< isoproterenol), and hypertension. Drug bolus can cause severe hypertension and marked peripheral vasoconstriction with no capillary refill.

Doses > 20 mcg/kg/minute can cause arrhythmias, decreased cardiac output, increased myocardial O_2 consumption, increased systemic and pulmonary vascular resistance.

Can cause tissue necrosis with extravasation.

Use with caution in infants with heart disease, pulmonary hypertension, or liver dysfunction.

Solution Compatibility

D5W, D10W, 0.9% NaCl.

Additive Compatibility

Dobutamine, heparin, lidocaine, potassium chloride.

Additive Incompatibility

Amphotericin B.

Drug Interactions

Phenytoin: pharmacologic action of dopamine may be decreased. Severe hypotension and bradycardia may occur with administration of phenytoin IV.

Nursing Considerations

- Quick solution dilution: # **mg** of dopamine to add to 100 ml IV solution = weight

(kg) × # mcg/kg/minute ×
6, at infusion rate of 1 ml/
hour.

If volume of drug to be added to 100 ml IV solution
is > 10 ml (> 10% of total volume), adjust IV solution volume so total volume equals 100 ml.

- Stop or decrease infusion rate if undesired effects
  occur.
- Double-check dose and rate of infusion.
- Maintain continuous IV infusion. Use controlled infu-
  sion device for administration.
- Use large vein for administration.
- Observe IV site closely for extravasation. Treatment
  for extravasation: Phentolamine (Regitine) 0.5 mg/ml
  0.9% NaCl. Infiltrate throughout affected area as
  soon as possible. Use 25 gauge needle.
- Blanching due to local vasoconstriction may be nor-
  mally observed along vein.
- Monitor HR, rhythm, and arterial BP continuously.
- Assess capillary refill.
- Monitor for adequate oxygenation, ventilation, and
  acid-base balance: (blood gases, TcO_2, $TcCO_2$, O_2
  saturation).
- Caution when changing solution daily (avoid bolus
  or prolonged interruption of drug infusion). Monitor
  closely for changes in BP.
- Do NOT BOLUS other drugs via dopamine infusion.
- Monitor urine output.
- Monitor serum sodium.
- Refrigerate open vial. Discard after 24 hours.
- Stable for 24 hours after dilution with a compatible
  IV solution.

Epinephrine

Brand Names

Adrenalin, various

Forms

Injection 1 mg/10 ml (0.1 mg/ml) 1:10,000 dilution.
1 mg/1 ml 1:1,000 dilution.

Uses

Cardiopulmonary resuscitation for the treatment of asystole or bradycardia despite adequate ventilation and cardiac compressions.
Improvement of cardiac output and blood pressure in cardiogenic shock states refractory to dopamine and/or dobutamine. Short-term use.
Enhances electrical defibrillation in the presence of ventricular fibrillation.

Dose

Cardiopulmonary Resuscitation.   0.01 mg/kg/dose (0.1 ml/kg of **1:10,000**) IV, ET, IC q 5 minutes prn. Provide adequate ventilation and cardiac compressions and correct hypovolemia prior to administration. Drug is ineffective if pH is < 7.10.
Cardiogenic Shock.   0.05–1 mcg/kg/minute. Continuous IV infusion.
Start with low dose (0.05–0.1 mcg/kg/minute) and titrate to desired effect.
Correct hypovolemia and acidosis prior to administration. Drug is ineffective if pH is < 7.10.

   Increases myocardial contractility, heart rate, blood

pressure (systolic and diastolic), systemic vascular resistance, myocardial O_2 consumption; decreases blood flow to kidneys. Decreases peripheral vascular resistance at low doses.

Pharmacokinetics

Onset of action is immediate after IV administration. Peak effect occurs between 1–2 minutes. Rapid onset of action after ET administration. Rapidly metabolized in the liver and other tissues. Small amounts are excreted unchanged in the urine.

Cautions

Can cause tachycardia, arrhythmias, severe hypertension with cerebral hemorrhage, renal vascular ischemia, hypokalemia, and hyperglycemia. Hyperglycemia is caused by inhibition of insulin secretion.

Hazards of IC administration include: pneumothorax, hemopericardium, coronary artery laceration, myocardial necrosis (with injection of drug into the myocardium), and irreversible ventricular arrhythmia.

Can cause tissue necrosis with extravasation after IV administration.

Solution Compatibility

Dextrose-saline combinations, D5W, D10W, 0.9% NaCl.

Additive Compatibility

Dobutamine.

Drug Interactions

Isoproterenol: simultaneous administration with epinephrine may produce serious arrhythmia due to combined effect.

Propranolol: effects such as increased systolic and diastolic blood pressure, marked decrease in heart rate, and epinephrine resistance may occur.

Tolazoline: large doses of tolazoline administered concurrently with epinephrine may cause a paradoxical fall in BP followed by an exaggerated rebound increase in BP.

Nursing Considerations

- Use 1 mg/10 ml (**1:10,000**) dilution for CPR (bolus administration).
- Use IC route only in infant without ET or IV access.
- Use 1 mg/ml (1:1,000) dilution to prepare continuous IV infusion.
- Quick solution dilution: **# mg** of epinephrine to add to 100 ml IV solution = weight (kg) × # mcg/kg/minute × 6, at infusion rate of 1 ml/hour.

  If volume of drug to be added to 100 ml IV solution is > 10 ml (> 10% of total volume), adjust IV solution volume so total volume equals 100 ml.
- Stop or decrease infusion rate if undesired effects occur.
- Dougle-check dose and rate of infusion.
- Maintain continuous IV infusion. Use controlled infusion device for administration.
- Caution when changing solution daily (avoid bolus

or prolonged interruption of drug infusion). Monitor closely for changes in BP.
- Use large vein for administration.
- Observe IV site closely for extravasation. Treatment for extravasation: Phentolamine (Regitine) 0.5 mg/ml 0.9% NaCl. Infiltrate throughout ischemic area as soon as possible. Use 25 gauge needle.
- Monitor HR, rhythm, and arterial BP continuously.
- Assess peripheral pulses and capillary refill.
- Monitor for adequate oxygenation, ventilation, and acid-base balance: (blood gases, TcO_2, $TcCO_2$, O_2 saturation).
- Do NOT BOLUS other drugs via epinephrine infusion.
- Monitor urine output.
- Monitor serum potassium and blood glucose.
- Do not use if color or precipitate present.
- Protect from light.

Isoproterenol

Brand Name

Isuprel

Forms

Injection 1 mg/5 ml (200 mcg/ml) 1:5000 dilution.

Uses

Improvement of cardiac output in cardiogenic shock states.

Dose

0.05–1 mcg/kg/minute. Continuous IV infusion.
Start with low dose (0.05–0.1 mcg/kg/minute) and
titrate to desired effect.
Correct hypovolemia and acidosis prior to administration.

Increases myocardial contractility, HR (> dopamine
and dobutamine), and myocardial O_2 consumption;
decreases systemic and peripheral vascular resistance with decreased or unchanged blood pressure
and blood flow to kidneys. .

Pharmacokinetics

Onset of action is immediate. Duration of action is < 1
hour. Fifty percent is excreted unchanged in the urine;
25–35% is metabolized in the liver to an active metabolite with weak β-blocker activity (metabolite has short
half-life).

Cautions

Can cause tachycardia, arrhythmias, myocardial
necrosis, hypotension, and hypoglycemia. Hypoglycemia is caused by increased secretion of insulin due
to increased glycogenesis effect of drug.

Use with caution in infants with kidney dysfunction,
preexisting arrhythmias, or digoxin toxicity.

Solution Compatibility

Dextrose-saline combinations, D5W, D10W, 0.45%
NaCl, 0.9% NaCl.

Additive Compatibility

Dobutamine, heparin, magnesium sulfate, potassium chloride.

Additive Incompatibility

Lidocaine.

Drug Interactions

Epinephrine: simultaneous administration with isoproterenol may produce serious arrhythmia due to combined effect.

Nursing Considerations

- Quick solution dilution: **#** **mg** of isoproterenol to add to 100 ml IV solution = weight (kg) × # mcg/kg/minute × 6, at infusion rate of 1 ml/hour.

  If volume of drug to be added to 100 ml IV solution is > 10 ml (> 10% of total volume), adjust IV solution volume so total volume equals 100 ml.
- Stop or decrease infusion rate if undesired effects occur.
- Double-check dose and rate of infusion.
- Maintain continuous IV infusion. Use controlled infusion device for administration.
- Monitor HR, rhythm, arterial BP, and CVP continuously.
- Monitor for adequate oxygenation, ventilation, and acid-base balance: (blood gases, TcO_2, $TcCO_2$, O_2 saturation).
- Do NOT bolus other drugs via isoproterenol infusion.

- Monitor blood glucose.
- Do not use if color or precipitate present.
- Stable at room temperature.

Other CV Drugs

Alprostadil (PGE₁)

Alprostadil (PGE$_1$)

Brand Name

Prostin VR Pediatric

Forms

Injection 500 mcg/ml.

Uses

Maintains temporary patency of the ductus arteriosus (DA) in infants with treatable ductus-dependent cyanotic and acyanotic heart lesions, until palliative or corrective surgery can be performed.
Cyanotic lesions include: pulmonary atresia, severe pulmonary stenosis, tricuspid, atresia, tetralogy of Fallot, and transposition of the great vessels.
Acyanotic lesions include: severe coarctation of the aorta, interruption of the aortic arch, and severe aortic stenosis.

Dose

Initial dose: 0.05–0.1 mcg/kg/minute. Continuous IV infusion. Maximum dose is 0.4 mcg/kg/minute (higher doses do not increase efficacy).
Decrease dose once patency of the DA has been

established (increased pO_2 or TcO_2 > 10 torr, increased O_2 saturation, palpable femoral pulses, improved lower extremity perfusion, increased urine output).

Maintenance: 0.01–0.05 mcg/kg/minute can be effective in maintaining patency of the DA.

Pharmacokinetics

Maximum effect is seen within 15–30 minutes with cyanotic heart lesions; within 1.5–3 hours with acyanotic lesions. Half-life is 5–10 minutes, necessitating continuous IV infusion. Duration of effect is 1–2 hours after infusion is discontinued (closure of the DA usually begins at this time). Metabolized rapidly in the lungs with metabolites excreted in the urine.

Cautions

Side effects by body systems include:

CV: flushing, edema, hypotension, bradycardia, tachycardia, arrhythmias, precipitation or aggravation of congestive heart failure, cardiac arrest.

CNS: fever, irritability, jitteriness, lethargy, seizure-like activity.

Respiratory: respiratory depression, apnea (most common in infants < 2 kg and during the first hours of administration).

GI: diarrhea, necrotizing enterocolitis (rare), hyperbilirubinemia (rare).

Renal: renal insufficiency or failure.

Metabolic: hypoglycemia, hypokalemia.

Hematologic: decreased platelet function, thrombocytopenia, DIC, hemorrhage.

Side effects are most common in infants with cyanotic heart lesions, infants < 2 kg weight, and infants receiving drug infusion > 48 hours.

Long-term use can cause damage to the DA with possible aneurysm formation and ductal rupture.

Use with caution in infants with pulmonary disease.

Solution Compatibility

D5W, 0.9% NaCl.

Additive Compatibility

Do NOT mix with other drugs.

Nursing Considerations

- Quick solution dilution: **# mcg** of alprostadil to add to 100 ml IV solution = weight (kg) × # mcg/kg/minute × 6 × 1000 at infusion rate of 1 ml/hour.

  If volume of drug to be added to 1000 ml IV solution is > 10 ml (> 10% of total volume), adjust IV solution volume so total volume equals 100 ml.
- Maintain continuous IV infusion. Use controlled infusion device for administration.
- Do not bolus other drugs via alprostadil infusion.
- Have means of assisted ventilation at bedside.
- Have IV fluid bolus at bedside.
- Monitor HR, rhythm, BP, respiratory effort, and temperature continuously. Assess femoral pulses and upper and lower extremity BPs in infants with left-sided obstructive lesions.
- Assess infant's response to drug (improvement in oxygenation and perfusion). Monitor blood gases,

continuous TcO$_2$, TcCO$_2$ and/or O$_2$ saturation, and
assess capillary refill.
- Assess infant's activity.
- Monitor platelet count and blood glucose.
- Monitor kidney function and urine output.
- Stable in solution for 24 hours.
- Refrigerate drug.
- Osmolality (Prostin VR Pediatric 500 mcg/ml):
  23,250 mOsm/kg H$_2$O (FP).

Atropine

Brand Names

Various

Forms

Injection 400 mcg/ml, 1 mg/ml, 1 mg/10 ml (may contain benzyl alcohol or parabens).

Uses

Treatment of vagally mediated bradycardia (e.g., intubation attempts).
Treatment of sinus bradycardia with 2° or 3° heart block.
Reduces muscarinic effects of neostigmine when reversing neuromuscular blockade.

Dose

0.01 mg/kg/dose (0.1 ml/kg of 1 mg/10 ml dilution) IV, ET q 10–15 minutes.
Maximum total dose 0.04 mg/kg.
   Increases heart rate and atrioventricular (AV) conduction; decreases vagal tone.

Pharmacokinetics

Rapid onset of action after IV or ET administration. Peak effect occurs between 2 and 5 minutes. Duration of action up to 6 hours. Half-life is 2–3 hours. Primarily excreted unchanged in the urine.

Cautions

Can cause mild transient bradycardia, tachycardia, arrhythmias (during first 2 minutes after administration), increased myocardial O_2 consumption, CNS depression (dose dependent), flushing, fever, esophageal reflux (due to decreased sphincter tone), and abdominal distention (due to decreased bowel activity). Causes pupil dilation. Lower doses more likely to cause arrhythmias than large doses in infants.

Use with caution in infants with myocardial ischemia.

Solution Compatibility

D5W, 0.9% NaCl.

Additive Compatibility

Cimetidine, fentanyl, meperidine, metoclopramide, morphine.

Nursing Considerations

- Infuse slowly IV push over 1 minute.
- Observe infant's response to drug.
- Monitor HR and rhythm continuously.
- Monitor for adequate oxygenation, ventilation, and acid-base balance: (blood gases, TcO_2, $TcCO_2$, O_2 saturation).

- Assess level of consciousness.
- Observe for abdominal distention. Check bowel sounds.
- Observe for upper airway obstruction due to esophageal reflux. Suction prn.
- Monitor infant's temperature.

Digoxin

Brand Names

Lanoxin, various

Forms

Pediatric injection 100 mcg/ml (contains propylene glycol and alcohol).
Elixir 50 mcg/ml (contains propylene glycol and alcohol).

Uses

Treatment of congestive heart failure (CHF) due to decreased myocardial contractility.
Antiarrhythmic. Drug of choice for supraventricular arrhythmias, especially paroxysmal atrial tachycardia.

Dose

Total Digitalizing Dose (TDD)	Maintenance Dose
Preterm 10–20 mcg/kg IV, PO.	5–8 mcg/kg/day IV, PO q 12–24 hours.
Term 30–40 mcg/kg IV, PO.	10 mcg/kg/day IV, PO q 12 hours.
> 1 month 40 mcg/kg IV, PO.	10–15 mcg/kg/day IV, PO q 12 hours.

Cardiovascular (CV) Drugs

TDD is administered in divided doses at 8 hour intervals (1/2 TDD × 1, then 1/4 TDD × 2). Start maintenance 24 hours after digitalization in the pre-term infant, 12 hours in the term and older infant.
For slow digitalization: begin maintenance dose, digitalization will be complete in 5–7 days.
Decrease dose in infants with kidney dysfunction.

   Improves myocardial contractility. Decreases myocardial excitability and conduction. Increases vagal tone.

   ECG effects include: increased PR and decreased QT intervals.

   Hemodynamic effects include: increased BP ($\pm$) and cardiac output.

Pharmacokinetics

Onset of action is 5–30 minutes after IV administration; 1–2 hours after PO administration. Rapidly and well absorbed from the GI tract after PO administration (~80%). Food delays absorption. Half-life is 15–72 hours (mean). Clearance increases with maturation of kidney function over the first weeks of life. Mostly excreted unchanged in the urine (60%) with metabolites; 40% is metabolized in the liver and intestines to inactive metabolites.
Therapeutic serum concentration: 2–4 ng/ml. Serum drug concentration does not always correlate well with efficacy or toxicity of the drug.

Cautions

Toxicity can cause bradycardia or arrest, arrhythmias (sinus bradycardia, ventricular tachycardia), conduction disturbances (2° or 3° heart block), and precipitation or aggravation of CHF. Can also cause drowsiness, lethargy, weakness, seizures (rare), poor feeding, vomiting, failure to thrive, and weight loss.

Factors that can precipitate toxicity (even at recommended doses) include: prematurity, hypoxemia, hypokalemia (common with concomitant diuretic administration), hypomagnesemia, hypercalcemia, metabolic acidosis, myocarditis, or severe liver or kidney dysfunction.

Use with caution in infants with kidney or liver dysfunction.

Solution Compatibility

D5W, 0.9% NaCl, TPN (compatible with most IV solutions).

Additive Compatibility

Do NOT mix with other drugs.

Drug Interactions

Antacids: decrease absorption of digoxin from the GI tract.
Furosemide: frequency of cardiac arrhythmias due to digoxin may be increased.
Hydrochlorothiazide: see "*Furosemide.*"
Metoclopramide: effects of oral digoxin may be decreased.
Quinidine: toxic effects of digoxin may be increased due to increased serum digoxin levels, while inotropic action may be decreased.
Verapamil: increases digoxin serum concentrations 50–75%.

Cardiovascular (CV) Drugs

Nursing Considerations

- CAUTION: dead space in syringe (hub) is significantly greater than intended dose. DO NOT FLUSH SYRINGE AFTER ADMINISTRATION.
- Double-check, with another nurse, dose/volume drawn up in syringe prior to administration.
- Obtain infant's HR for a full minute prior to administration and record.
- Infuse slowly IV push over 5 minutes.
- Do not administer IM (can cause pain and local tissue necrosis), absorption is erratic.
- Administer PO preparation on an empty stomach if possible.
- Obtain a 12-lead ECG prior to the start of digitalization.
- Obtain lead 2 rhythm strip prior to each digitalizing dose and prior to the first maintenance dose and as indicated thereafter. Measure PR interval. Normal PR interval is 0.07–0.14 seconds.
- Monitor HR and rhythm.
- Monitor blood gases (pH, pCO_2, pO_2, base deficit).
- Observe for signs of heart failure: respiratory distress (tachypnea, retractions, wheezing, grunting, flaring), tachycardia, gallop rhythm, peripheral cyanosis, metabolic acidosis, liver enlargement, sweating, lethargy or irritability, restlessness, poor feeding, and failure to thrive.
- Observe infant's response to drug: decreased respiratory distress, normal HR and rhythm, decreased irritability, improved feeding, and weight gain.
- Serum drug concentrations are not needed routinely

if infant is stable and there are no signs of toxicity (routine measurements can be important as the infant grows). If a serum concentration is indicated, obtain blood 6–8 hours after a dose or just before a dose.

- Monitor kidney function, serum potassium, and calcium.
- Provide parents with written instructions for administering digoxin (see Appendix D: Drug Information for Parents).
- Osmolality (Lanoxin elixir 50 mcg/ml) 4480 mOsm/kg H_2O (FP).
  (Lanoxin injection 100 mcg/ml): 9105 mOsm/kg H_2O (FP).

Treatment for Digoxin-Induced Arrhythmias:

Phenytoin. Drug of choice for digoxin-induced atrial and ventricular arrhythmias.
2–5 mg/kg/dose over 5–10 minutes (to maximum initial dose of 20 mg/kg).
Lidocaine. Atrial and ventricular arrhythmias.
1 mg/kg/dose over 5–10 minutes (to maximum initial dose of 5 mg/kg).
Atropine. Sinus bradycardia and 2° or 3° heart block.
0.01 mg/kg/dose (up to maximum dose of 0.04 mg/kg).

Indomethacin

Brand Name

Indocin

Forms

1 mg for IV use only (for reconstitution).

Uses

Closure of hemodynamically significant patent ductus arteriosus (PDA).

Dose

Age	1st dose	2nd dose	3rd dose
< 48 hours	0.2 mg/kg IV	0.1 mg/kg IV	0.1 mg/kg IV
> 48 hours	0.2 mg/kg IV	0.2 mg/kg IV	0.2 mg/kg IV
> 1 week	0.2 mg/kg IV	0.2 mg/kg IV	0.2 mg/kg IV

Doses are administered at 12 hour intervals. Maximum dose is 0.6 mg/kg in a 36 hour period. Maximum three doses per "course." Maximum two "courses." Administration of subsequent doses should be based on persistence of the PDA.

Pharmacokinetics

Poor and incomplete absorption from the GI tract of the preterm infant after PO administration of available oral suspension (~20% bioavailable). Half-life is variable, 15–50 hours (mean 30 hours). Clearance increases with postnatal age. Metabolized in the liver to inactive metabolites and excreted in the urine and bile. Small amounts are excreted unchanged in the urine. Highly plasma protein bound.
Therapeutic serum concentration: 0.2–0.8 mcg/ml.

Cautions

Causes decreased renal blood flow with transient and reversible kidney dysfunction (decreased urine output, decreased Na, Cl, and K excretion, decreased creatinine clearance with increased serum creatinine and BUN). Decreases GI blood flow with possible transient ileus, abdominal distention, GI bleeding, focal GI ulceration or perforation, and necrotizing enterocolitis. Decreases platelet function and prolongs bleeding time with possible pulmonary hemorrhage, DIC, and risk of precipitation or extension of an intraventricular hemorrhage. Can also cause hypoglycemia, hyponatremia, and hyperkalemia. Preliminary studies show it decreases cerebral blood flow velocity as much as 50% (persisting up to 1 hour) when drug is administered at the recommended infusion rate of 2 minutes.

Contraindications for drug administration include:
– BUN ≥ 30 mg/dl.
– serum creatinine ≥ 1.8 mg/dl.
– urine output ≤ 0.5–0.6 ml/kg/hour over past 8–12 hours.
– platelet count ≤ 50,000–60,000/mm^3.
– stools positive for occult blood.
– evidence of active bleeding.
– clinical and/or radiographic evidence of necrotizing enterocolitis.
– evidence of intraventricular hemorrhage in past 24–48 hours.

Solution Compatibility

Further dilution of reconstituted drug in IV solutions is not recomended.

Additive Compatibility

Do NOT mix with other drugs.

Cardiovascular (CV) Drugs   **99**

Drug Interactions

Captopril: antihypertensive effectiveness of captopril may be decreased or completely abolished, particularly in low-renin hypertension.

Furosemide: diuretic effect of furosemide may be decreased. Furosemide is often used during indomethacin therapy to maintain adequate urine output.

Propranolol: antihypertensive effect of propranolol may be decreased.

Nursing Considerations

- Infuse slowly IV over 2 minutes.
- Use vein for IV administration. Administration of drug through a UAC may result in a bolus to the renal arteries.
- Assess for presence of a PDA. Clinical signs of a PDA include:
  - hyperactive precordium.
  - bounding peripheral pulses.
  - widened pulse pressure ($\geq$ 35 mm Hg).
  - respiratory distress (tachypnea, hypercapnia, rales, need for increased respiratory support).
  - murmur (over left midclavicular line).
  - enlarged liver ($\geq$ 3 cm below the costal margin).
- Monitor kidney function (BUN and creatinine) and urine output. Obtain serum BUN and creatinine prior to each dose.
- Monitor platelet count. Obtain platelet count prior to each dose.
- Monitor serum electrolytes and glucose.
- Monitor GI function (measure abdominal girth,

assess bowel sounds, check gastric secretions and stools for occult blood).
- Observe for prolonged bleeding from puncture sites.
- Reconstituted drug is stable for 24 hours refrigerated.

Chapter 4

Neuromuscular (NM) Drugs

Skeletal Muscle Relaxants

Atracurium

Brand Name

Tracurium

Forms

Injection 10 mg/ml.

Uses

Skeletal muscle relaxant (nondepolarizing). Paralysis of short duration for intubation or a test dose to assess efficacy of muscle paralysis during mechanical ventilation of infant. Adjunct to general anesthesia.

Dose

0.1 mg/kg/dose IV.

Pharmacokinetics

Onset of action is within 30 seconds to 2 minutes. Peak effect occurs between 3 and 5 minutes. Duration of action is 20–30 minutes. Largely metabolized in the plasma; <10% is excreted unchanged in the bile.

Totally independent of liver and kidney function for elimination.

Cautions

Rapid IV infusion can cause tachycardia, hypotension, bronchospasm, increased bronchial secretions, flushing and erythema due to histamine release. Cardiovascular effects are minimal at suggested dose and increase with increased dose or frequency of administration.

Solution Compatibility

D5W, 0.9% NaCl.

Additive Compatibility

Do NOT mix with other drugs.

Drug Interactions

Aminoglycosides (amikacin, gentamicin, tobramycin): neuromuscular blocking effects of nondepolarizing muscle relaxants may be increased. Prolonged respiratory depression with extended periods of apnea may occur.
Aminophylline/theophylline: possible resistance to, or reversal of, the neuromuscular blocking effects of nondepolarizing muscle relaxants (theophylline dose dependent).
Clindamycin: see "*Aminoglycosides.*"
Halothane (general anesthetics): see "*Aminoglycosides.*"
Magnesium sulfate: see "*Aminoglycosides.*"

Nursing Considerations

- Infuse slowly IV push over 1 minute.
- Have intubation setup ready.
- Provide ventilatory support and oxygen delivery.
- Monitor for adequate oxygenation and ventilation (blood gases, TcO_2, $TcCO_2$, O_2 saturation, color).
- Reversal of nondepolarizing blockade: NEOSTIGMINE 0.06 mg/kg and ATROPINE 0.02 mg/kg (atropine is administered with neostigmine to minimize bradycardia, bronchospasm, increased salivation). Peak effect is within 5–10 minutes.
- Monitor HR and BP.
- Maintain patent airway; suction prn.
- Drug does not affect consciousness or pain threshold.
- Potentiation of drug effect occurs with acidosis, younger age, hypothermia, neuromuscular disease, cardiovascular disease, hypokalemia, hypocalcemia, hypermagnesemia, or use of other skeletal muscle relaxants.
- Antagonism of drug occurs with alkalosis, older age, or hyperkalemia.
- Refrigerate drug.

Pancuronium

Brand Name

Pavulon

Forms

Injection 1 mg/ml, 2 mg/ml (contains benzyl alcohol).

Uses

Skeletal muscle relaxant (nondepolarizing). Voluntary muscle paralysis during mechanical ventilation of infant. Adjunct to general anesthesia.

Dose

0.05–0.1 mg/kg/dose IV prn to maintain paralysis. Increase dose if duration of paralysis is <2–3 hours. Decrease dose if duration of paralysis is >4–6 hours.

Pharmacokinetics

Onset of action is within 1–2 minutes. Peak effect occurs between 4–5 minutes. Duration of action is 30–60 minutes. Less than 50% of drug is metabolized; 40% is excreted unchanged in the urine and 10% is excreted unchanged in the bile. Significant protein binding may occur.

Cautions

Can cause erythema, tachycardia, and a slight increase in blood pressure. Increased HR and BP may be due to vagolytic or sympathomimetic effect.

Rapid IV infusion can cause tachycardia, hypotension, bronchospasm, increased bronchial secretions, flushing, and erythema possibly due to histamine release.

Use with caution in infants with liver or kidney dysfunction.

Solution Compatibility

D5W, 0.9% NaCl.

Additive Compatibility

Do NOT mix with other drugs.

Drug Interactions

See "Drug Interactions" of atracurium.
Phenytoin: possible resistance to, or reversal of, the neuromuscular blocking effects of nondepolarizing muscle relaxants.

Nursing Considerations

- Infuse slowly IV push over 1 minute.
- Use ONLY if infant is on ventilator.
- Have bag and mask ventilation setup at bedside in case of ventilator malfunction or failure.
- Have intubation setup at bedside in case of "accidental" extubation.
- Monitor for adequate oxygenation and ventilation (blood gases, TcO_2, $TcCO_2$, O_2 saturation, color).
- Reversal of nondepolarizing blockade: NEOSTIGMINE 0.06 mg/kg and ATROPINE 0.02 mg/kg (atropine is administered with neostigmine to minimize bradycardia, bronchospasm, increased salivation). Peak effect is within 5–10 minutes.
- Monitor HR and BP.
- Maintain patent airway; suction prn.
- Drug does not affect consciousness or pain threshold. Provide sedation or analgesia as indicated by infant's clinical status.
- Assess infant's need for sedation or analgesia:
  – intolerance of handling and/or care.
  – change in vital signs (increased HR, BP).
  – decreased TcO_2 and/or O_2 saturation, increased $TcCO_2$.

- Observe infant for movement and tolerance of movement.
- Change infant's position as tolerated.
- Perform passive range of motion as tolerated.
- Potentiation of drug effect occurs with acidosis, younger age, hypothermia, neuromuscular disease, cardiovascular disease, liver or kidney dysfunction, hypokalemia, hypocalcemia, hypermagnesemia, or use of other skeletal muscle relaxants.
- Antagonism of drug effect occurs with alkalosis, older age, or hyperkalemia.
- Monitor liver and kidney function.
- Do not store drug in plastic container or syringe. Drug may be absorbed by plastics. Drug may be administered in plastic syringe.
- Refrigerate drug.

Succinylcholine

Brand Names

Anectine, various

Forms

Injection 20 mg/ml, 50 mg/ml.

Uses

Skeletal muscle relaxant (depolarizing). Rapid paralysis of short duration for intubation.

Dose

1–2 mg/kg/dose IV.
3–4 mg/kg/dose IM.

Neuromuscular (NM) Drugs   **107**

Pharmacokinetics

Onset of action is <1 minute after IV administration; 2–3 minutes after IM administration. Duration of action is 4–6 minutes IV; 10–30 minutes IM. Rapidly metabolized, largely in the plasma, to a metabolite with weak nondepolarizing activity; 10% is excreted unchanged in the urine. Histamine release is weak.

Cautions

Can cause bradycardia, increased or decreased BP, arrhythmias, sinus arrest (due to vagal stimulation), increased salivation, hyperthermia, and hyperkalemia. Tachyphylaxis with repeated doses. Continuous administration over a prolonged period can result in irreversible blockade.

Use with caution in infants with hyperkalemia (drug can cause the release of intracellular potassium).

Use with caution in infants with liver or kidney dysfunction.

Solution Compatibility

Dextrose-saline combinations, D5W, D10W, 0.45% NaCl, 0.9% NaCl.

Additive Compatibility

Amikacin, isoproterenol, meperidine, morphine.

Additive Incompatibility

Nafcillin, phenobarbital, sodium bicarbonate.

Drug Interactions

Aminoglycosides (amikacin, gentamicin, tobramycin): neuromuscular blocking effects of succinylcholine may be increased. Prolonged respiratory depression with extended periods of apnea may occur.

Cimetidine: see "*Aminoglycosides.*"
Lidocaine: see "*Aminoglycosides*" (dose dependent).
Neostigmine: see "*Aminoglycosides.*"

Nursing Considerations

- Have intubation setup ready.
- Provide ventilatory support and oxygen delivery.
- Monitor for adequate oxygenation and ventilation (blood gases, TcO_2, $TcCO_2$, O_2 saturation, color).
- Monitor HR, rhythm, and BP.
- Maintain patent airway; suction prn.
- NO known antagonist for the reversal of depolarizing blockade.
- Drug does not affect consciousness or pain threshold.
- Potentiation of drug effect occurs with alkalosis, hypokalemia, or hypothermia.
- Antagonism of drug effect occurs with acidosis.
- Monitor serum potassium.
- Refrigerate drug.

Vecuronium

Brand Name

Norcuron

Forms

Injection 10 mg vial (powder for reconstitution) (contains benzyl alcohol).

Neuromuscular (NM) Drugs

Uses

Skeletal muscle relaxant (nondepolarizing). Voluntary muscle paralysis during mechanical ventilation of infant. Adjunct to general anesthesia.

Dose

0.05–0.1 mg/kg/dose IV prn to maintain paralysis. Increase dose if duration of paralysis is <2–3 hours. Decrease dose if duration of paralysis is >4–6 hours.

Pharmacokinetics

Onset of action is within 2–3 minutes. Peak effect occurs between 3–5 minutes. Duration of action is 25–60 minutes. Some drug is metabolized in the liver to an active metabolite and excreted in the bile and urine. Largely excreted unchanged in the urine.

Cautions

Rapid IV infusion can cause tachycardia, hypotension, bronchospasm, increased bronchial secretions, flushing and erythema possibly due to histamine release.

Use with caution in infants with liver or kidney dysfunction.

Solution Compatibility

D5W, 0.9% NaCl.

Additive Compatibility

Do NOT mix with other drugs.

Drug Interactions

See "Drug Interactions" of atracurium.
Phenytoin: possible resistance to, or reversal of, the neuromuscular blocking effects of nondepolarizing muscle relaxants.

Nursing Considerations

- Infuse slowly IV push over 1 minute.
- Use ONLY if infant is on ventilator.
- Have bag and mask ventilation setup at bedside in case of ventilator malfunction or failure.
- Have intubation setup at bedside in case of "accidental" extubation.
- Monitor for adequate oxygenation and ventilation (blood gases, TcO_2, $TcCO_2$, O_2 saturation, color).
- Reversal of nondepolarizing blockade: NEOSTIGMINE 0.06 mg/kg and ATROPINE 0.02 mg/kg (atropine is administered with neostigmine to minimize bradycardia, bronchospasm, increased salivation). Peak effect is within 5–10 minutes.
- Monitor HR and BP.
- Maintain patent airway; suction prn.
- Drug does not affect consciousness or pain threshold. Provide sedation or analgesia as indicated by infant's clinical status.
- Assess infant's need for sedation or analgesia:
  – intolerance of handling and/or care.
  – change in vital signs (increased HR, BP).
  – decreased TcO_2 and/or O_2 saturation, increased $TcCO_2$.
- Observe infant for movement and tolerance of movement.

Neuromuscular (NM) Drugs　　　　　　　**111**

- Change infant's position as tolerated.
- Perform passive range of motion as tolerated.
- Potentiation of drug effect occurs with acidosis, younger age, hypothermia, neuromuscular disease, cardiovascular disease, liver or kidney dysfunction, hypokalemia, hypocalcemia, hypermagnesemia, or use of other skeletal muscle relaxants.
- Antagonism of drug effect occurs with alkalosis, older age, or hyperkalemia.
- Monitor liver and kidney function.
- Refrigerate reconstituted drug.
- Stable for 24 hours after reconstitution if refrigerated.

Chapter 5

Renal Drugs

Diuretics

Furosemide

Brand Names

Lasix, various

Forms

Injection 20 mg/2 ml.
Oral solution 10 mg/ml (contains alcohol).

Uses

Potent diuretic. Treatment of fluid overload state of any etiology (i.e., CHF, RDS, PDA, and BPD).

Dose

Initial dose: 1 mg/kg/dose IV, IM, PO.
Maximum dose: 2 mg/kg/dose IV, IM, and 6 mg/kg/dose PO.
Frequency of administration should be based on diuretic response and clinical status of the infant: preterm q 24 hours, term q 12 hours, >1 month q 6–8 hours.

Pharmacokinetics

Onset of action is within 20–60 minutes after IV administration, with peak diuresis between 1 and 3 hours, and duration of action between 4 and 6 hours. Incomplete and variable absorption from the GI tract. Onset of action is within 1 hour after PO administration. Mean half-life is 8–27 hours (shorter in infants with low serum albumin). Clearance increases over the first month of life. Majority of the drug is excreted unchanged in the urine with inactive metabolites. Highly plasma protein bound.

Cautions

Can cause fluid and electrolyte imbalance (dehydration, hypovolemia with hypotension, hypokalemia, hyponatremia, hypochloremia), hypocalcemia, hyperglycemia, ototoxicity, and metabolic alkalosis with compensatory hypoventilation and hypercarbia. Increased risk of ototoxicity in infants with kidney dysfunction, with rapid IV infusion, or with concomitant administration of aminoglycosides. Increased risk of digoxin toxicity in hypokalemic infants. Drug can interfere with ductal closure by stimulating renal release of PGE_2.

Chronic therapy can cause kidney stones and gallstones; can also cause osteopenia (bone loss) with potential for rickets and fractures.

Use with caution in digitalized infants and infants with kidney dysfunction.

Solution Compatibility

D5W, D10W, D20W, 0.9% NaCl, TPN.

Additive Compatibility

Cimetidine, heparin.

Additive Incompatibility

Amikacin, dobutamine, epinephrine, gentamicin, tobramycin.

Drug Interactions

Aminoglycosides (amikacin, gentamicin, tobramycin): ototoxicity of both drugs may be increased.
Digoxin: possible increased frequency of cardiac arrhythmias due to digoxin.
Indomethacin: possible decreased diuretic effect of furosemide. Furosemide is often used during indomethacin therapy to maintain adequate urine output.

Nursing Considerations

- Infuse slowly IV push over 1–2 minutes.
- Administer PO preparation with feeding.
- Monitor urine output and kidney function.
- Weigh daily.
- Monitor serum electrolytes, calcium, phosphorus, and blood glucose.
- Observe/monitor for signs of dehydration: tachycardia, hypotension, depressed fontanelle, dry mucous membranes, poor skin turgor, decreased urine output (<2 ml/kg/hour).
- Observe/monitor for signs of fluid overload: increased respiratory distress, rales, peripheral edema, marked increase in weight.
- Attention to potential for fractures in infants on chronic therapy:
  - gentle handling and positioning.
  - gentle chest physiotherapy.
- Protect drug from light.

- Provide parents with written instructions for administering furosemide (see Appendix D: Drug Information for Parents).
- Osmolality (Lasix oral solution): 3580 mOsm/kg H_2O (FP).

Hydrochlorothiazide

Brand Names

HydroDIURIL, various

Forms

Tablets 25 mg, 50 mg (can be made into oral suspension).

Uses

Moderately potent diuretic. Treatment of mild to moderate fluid overload states (CHF, BPD, and kidney disease) and mild to moderate hypertension. Often used in combination with furosemide or spironolactone.

Dose

2–4 mg/kg/day PO q 12 hours. Adjust dose according to diuretic response and clinical status of infant. Increase dosing interval in infants with kidney failure.

Pharmacokinetics

Rapidly absorbed from the GI tract. Onset of action is within 1–2 hours, with peak diuresis between 2 and 6 hours, and duration of action between 6 and 12 hours. Half-life is up to 15 hours. Excreted unchanged in the urine with no metabolism of the drug. Moderately plasma protein bound.

Cautions

Can cause fluid and electrolyte imbalance (dehydration, hypokalemia, hyponatremia, hypochloremia), hypomagnesemia, hyperuricemia, glucose intolerance and hyperglycemia, and metabolic alkalosis with possible compensatory hypoventilation and hypercarbia. Increased risk of digoxin toxicity in infants with hypomagnesemia or hypokalemia. Can aggravate kidney or liver insufficiency. Can cause gastric irritation, vomiting, diarrhea, or constipation. Hypersensitivity can cause rash, photosensitivity, and bone marrow depression.

Use with caution in digitalized infants and in infants with kidney or liver dysfunction.

Drug Interactions

Digoxin: possible increased frequency of cardiac arrhythmias due to digoxin.

Nursing Considerations

• Administer with feeding (enhances absorption of drug).
• Shake suspension well before drawing up dose.
• Monitor urine output and daily weights.
• Monitor kidney and liver function.
• Monitor serum electrolytes, magnesium, and blood glucose.
• Observe/monitor for signs of dehydration: tachycardia, hypotension, depressed fontanelle, dry

mucous membranes, poor skin turgor, decreased urine output (<2 ml/kg/hour).

- Observe/monitor for signs of fluid overload: increased respiratory distress, rales, peripheral edema, marked increase in weight.
- Check with your pharmacy regarding stability of extemporaneously prepared suspension.

Hydrochlorothiazide and Spironolactone

Brand Name

Aldactazide

Forms

Tablets 25 mg hydrochlorothiazide and 25 mg spironolactone (can be made into oral suspension).

Uses

Moderately potent diuretic. Chronic treatment of fluid overload states (CHF, BPD).

Dose

1–3 mg/kg/day (of 1:1 suspension) PO q 12–24 hours. Adjust dose according to diuretic response and clinical status of infant.

Pharmacokinetics

Well absorbed from the GI tract. Onset of action is within 24 hours after initiation of treatment. Hydrochlorothiazide is excreted unchanged in the urine with no metabolism of the drug. Spironolactone is rapidly and completely metabolized in the liver to a large number of metabolites, which are excreted in the urine and bile. Moderate to highly plasma protein bound.

Cautions

Can cause fluid and electrolyte imbalance: dehydration, hypokalemia or hyperkalemia (dependent on kidney function), and hyponatremia. Can also cause gastric irritation, vomiting, and diarrhea. See also "Cautions" of the individual drugs.

Use with caution in digitalized infants and in infants with kidney or liver dysfunction.

Drug Interactions

Captopril: hyperkalemia may occur with possible cardiac arrhythmias or arrest.
Digoxin: possible increased frequency of cardiac arrhythmias due to digoxin.
Potassium preparations: see "*Captopril.*"

Nursing Considerations

- Administer with feeding (enhances absorption of drug).
- Shake suspension well before drawing up dose.
- Monitor urine output and daily weights.
- Monitor kidney and liver function.
- Monitor serum electrolytes.
- Observe/monitor for signs of dehydration: tachycardia, hypotension, depressed fontanelle, dry mucous membranes, poor skin turgor, decreased urine output (<2 ml/kg/hour).
- Observe/monitor for signs of fluid overload: increased respiratory distress, rales, peripheral edema, marked increase in weight.

- Check with your pharmacy regarding stability of extemporaneously prepared suspension.
- Provide parents with written instructions for administering Aldactazide (see Appendix D: Drug Information for Parents).

Spironolactone

Brand Name

Aldactone

Forms

Tablets 25 mg (can be made into oral suspension).

Uses

Moderately potent diuretic. Chronic treatment of fluid overload states associated with hyperaldosteronism (congenital heart disease and BPD). Often used in combination with hydrochlorothiazide.

Dose

1–3 mg/kg/day PO q 12–24 hours. Adjust dose according to diuretic response and clinical status of infant (3–5 days are required to evaluate response to drug due to its slow onset of action).

Pharmacokinetics

Onset of action is within 3–5 days after initiation of treatment. Diuresis may persist 2–3 days after the drug is discontinued. Rapidly and completely metabolized in the liver to a large number of metabolites (some active with substantially less activity than parent drug). Major active metabolite is canrenone with a half-life of 13–24 hours. Metabolites are excreted in the urine and bile. Highly plasma protein bound.

Cautions

"Potassium-sparing" diuretic, can cause hyperkalemia, with possible cardiac arrhythmias, especially in infants with kidney dysfunction or in infants receiving potassium supplements. Can also cause dehydration, hyponatremia, drowsiness, rash, gynecomastia, gastric irritation, vomiting, and diarrhea.

Use with caution in infants with liver or kidney dysfunction.

Drug Interactions

Captopril: hyperkalemia may occur with possible cardiac arrhythmias or arrest.

Potassium preparations: see "*Captopril.*"

Nursing Considerations

- Administer with feeding (enhances absorption of drug).
- Shake suspension well before drawing up dose.
- Monitor urine output and daily weights.
- Monitor kidney and liver function.
- Monitor serum electrolytes.
- Observe/monitor for signs of dehydration: tachycardia, hypotension, depressed fontanelle, dry

mucous membranes, poor skin turgor, decreased urine output (<2 ml/kg/hour).
- Observe/monitor for signs of fluid overload: increased respiratory distress, rales, peripheral edema, marked increase in weight.
- Check with your pharmacy regarding stability of extemporaneously prepared suspension.

Chapter 6

Gastrointestinal (GI) Drugs

Cimetidine

Brand Name

Tagamet

Forms

Injection 150 mg/ml in 2 and 4 ml vials (contains preservatives; may be made into a 1:10 dilution so small doses may be accurately measured).
Oral solution 60 mg/ml (contains alcohol 2.8% and preservatives).

Uses

H-2 antagonist. Treatment of duodenal, gastric or "stress" ulcers and upper GI bleeding.
Effectiveness of cimetidine prophylaxis to prevent GI ulceration/bleeding has not been proven. Simultaneous use of H-2 antagonists and antacids does not hasten ulcer healing.

Dose

5 mg/kg/dose IV, PO q 6 hours.
Daily dose may be added to infant's TPN solution and administered as a continuous infusion.

Pharmacokinetics

Rapidly and well absorbed from the GI tract after PO administration, with about 60–70% of the oral dose bioavailable. Presence of food will delay and possibly decrease absorption of drug. Widely distributed throughout tissues. Half-life is about 2.5 hours. Some metabolism in the liver with at least half the drug excreted unchanged in the urine along with metabolites. Small amounts excreted in the feces.
Accumulation of drug may occur in infants with severe kidney or liver impairment.
Serum concentrations of 0.5–1.0 mcg/ml result in reduction of gastric acidity by 50–90%.

Cautions

Adverse reactions are rare and usually mild. The most frequent reactions are mental confusion, disorientation, and headache, which cannot be assessed in infants. Agitation and restlessness or drowsiness can occur, as can mild diarrhea, rash, mild gynecomastia, and small transient increases of serum creatinine, SGOT, SGPT, and alkaline phosphatase. Rapid infusion may cause cardiac arrhythmias, bradycardia, and hypotension. May reduce hepatic blood flow resulting in increased half-life and increased effects of drugs metabolized in the liver.

   Use with caution in infants with liver or kidney dysfunction.

Solution Compatibility

D5W, 0.9% NaCl, TPN.

Additive Compatibility

Amikacin, clindamycin, dexamethasone, digoxin, furosemide, gentamicin, insulin, methylprednisolone, penicillin G, potassium chloride, vancomycin.

Additive Incompatibility

Atropine, amphotericin B, cefazolin.

Drug Interactions

Aminophylline/theophylline: effects of theophylline may be increased with possible increased theophylline plasma levels with toxicity (interaction not well documented in neonates).
Antacids: concurrent PO administration may result in reduced cimetidine absorption. Administer the drugs at least 1 hour apart.
Benzodiazepines (clonazepam, diazepam): effects of these drugs may be increased with possible excessive sedation.
Lidocaine: effects of lidocaine may be increased with possible increased plasma levels and toxicity.
Phenytoin: see "Lidocaine."
Procainamide: see "Lidocaine."
Propranolol: effects of propranolol may be increased with possible bradycardia and hypotension.
Quinidine: effects of quinidine may be increased with possible increased plasma levels with cardiac conduction disturbances and arrhythmias.
Succinylcholine: neuromuscular blocking effect of succinylcholine may be prolonged.

Nursing Considerations

- Infuse slowly IV over 15–20 minutes.
- Monitor HR, rhythm, and BP.
- Administer PO preparation during or after feeding.
- Monitor gastric pH.
- Monitor kidney and liver function.
- Observe infant for CNS effects (agitation, restlessness, or drowsiness).
- Observe infant for rash.

Metoclopramide

Brand Names

Reglan, various

Forms

Oral solution 1 mg/ml (contains preservatives).

Uses

Management of gastroesophageal reflux (increases tone of sphincter in lower esophagus and decreases gastric emptying time). Short-term use.

Dose

0.1 mg/kg/dose PO q 8 hours.

Pharmacokinetics

Rapidly and almost completely absorbed from the GI tract after PO administration. Variable bioavailability due to variable first-pass metabolism in the liver. Distribution of drug into tissues not presently established, though drug apparently penetrates the CNS to exert antinauseant activity (used in adult and pediatric patients receiving cancer chemotherapy). Onset of action is 30–60 minutes after PO administration. Exact metabolic fate has not been established. Probably only minimally metabolized with most of drug eliminated as unchanged and conjugated drug in the urine along with metabolites. It is not known if the metabolite is active. Correlation between serum levels and desired therapeutic effect has not been fully elucidated.

Cautions

Adverse reactions are infrequent at the low doses used to treat gastroesophageal reflux. Serious CNS adverse effects with high (antiemetic) doses (1–2 mg/kg) include restlessness, agitation, drowsiness, and extrapyramidal reactions (dystonic reactions include involuntary movements of the face and limbs, rhythmic protrusions of the tongue, opisthotonos, laryngospasms, and oculogyric crisis with deviation and fixation of eyeballs upward). The CNS effects may be reversed by administration of diphenhydramine (Benadryl) 0.5–1 mg/kg IV over 5 minutes. These adverse effects normally subside within 24 hours after discontinuing drug. Low doses used for the treatment of GE reflux (0.1 mg/kg) can cause drowsiness, constipation or diarrhea, and maculopapular rash.

Use with caution in infants with liver or kidney dysfunction.

CONTRAINDICATED in infants with a history of seizures, recent GI bleeding, or other GI disorders in which increased GI motility may exacerbate a preexisting condition (mechanical obstruction or perforation).

Drug Interactions

CNS depressants: depressant effect may be additive when used in combination with metoclopramide.
Digoxin: decreased digoxin serum levels with decreased digoxin effectiveness may occur. Decreased gastric emptying time due to metoclopramide use may result in incomplete gastric absorption of digoxin (or other drugs that are primarily absorbed in the stomach).
Opiates: constipating effects of narcotic analgesics may antagonize the increased GI motility induced by metoclopramide.

Nursing Considerations

- Administer 30 minutes before feedings.
- Observe infant for extrapyramidal signs: increased muscle tone, muscle rigidity, abnormal posturing, eyes rolled up or deviated to one side, rhythmic prostrusions of tongue.
- Observe for other CNS effects (restlessness, agitation, or drowsiness).
- Observe infant for rash.
- Assess effectiveness of drug. Observe for evidence of reflux ("spitting" to vomiting after feedings).
- Maintain infant in prone position at 30–45° angle, especially after feedings. Do NOT use infant seat.

Ranitidine

Brand Name

Zantac

Forms

Injection 25 mg/ml in 2 ml and 10 ml vials (contains preservative).
Oral solution 15 mg/ml.

Uses

H-2 antagonist. Treatment of duodenal, gastric or "stress" ulcers, and upper GI bleeding.
Effectiveness of ranitidine prophylaxis to prevent GI ulceration/bleeding has not been proven. Simultaneous use of H-2 antagonists and antacids does not hasten ulcer healing.

Dose

1–2 mg/kg/dose IV q 12 hours.
Daily dose may be added to infant's TPN solution and administered as a continuous infusion.
2–4 mg/kg/dose PO q 8 hours.

Pharmacokinetics

Rapidly and well absorbed from the GI tract after PO administration, with only about 50% of the oral drug bioavailable because of extensive first-pass metabolism in the liver. Widely distributed throughout tissues. Half-life is about 2 hours. Some metabolism in the liver with a large amount of an IV dose, and a smaller amount of a PO dose, excreted unchanged in the urine along with metabolites. Small amounts excreted in the feces. Accumulation of drug may occur in infants with kidney and liver dysfunction.

Cautions

Adverse reactions are rare and usually mild. The most frequent reactions are headache, dizziness, malaise, and mental confusion, which cannot be assessed in infants. Agitation or drowsiness can occur, as can constipation or diarrhea, vomiting, rash, painful gynecomastia, increases of serum creatinine (without increase in BUN), SGPT, SGOT, alkaline phosphatase, and rarely, tachycardia or bradycardia. May reduce hepatic blood flow resulting in increased half-life and increased effects of drugs metabolized in the liver.

Use with caution in infants with liver or kidney dysfunction.

Solution Compatibility

D5W, 0.9% NaCl, TPN.

Additive Compatibility

Atropine, fentanyl, metoclopramide, morphine.

Additive Incompatibility

Diazepam, phenobarbital.

Drug Interactions

Aminophylline/theophylline: effects of theophylline may be increased with possible increased theophylline plasma levels with toxicity.
Antacids: concurrent PO administration will result in

reduced ranitidine absorption. Administer the drugs at least 1 hour apart.

Diazepam: effects of diazepam may be increased with possible excessive sedation.

Propranolol: effects of propranolol may be increased with possible bradycardia and hypotension.

Nursing Considerations

- Infuse slowly IV over 15 minutes.
- Monitor gastric pH.
- Monitor kidney and liver function.
- Observe infant for CNS effects (agitation or drowsiness).
- Observe for rash.
- May cause false-positive result for protein in urine on Multistix.

Chapter 7

Anti-infectives

Antibiotics

AMINOGLYCOSIDES

Aminoglycosides are active against Gram-negative aerobic bacteria and some Gram-positive aerobic bacteria. Susceptible Gram-negative organisms include *Acinetobacter, Escherichia coli, Proteus mirabilis, Pseudomonas, Klebsiella, Enterobacter*, and *Serratia*. Susceptible Gram-positive organisms include *Staphylococcus aureus* and *Staphylococcus epidermidis*; these two organisms are rarely treated with an aminoglycoside as a sole agent.

Aminoglycosides are poorly absorbed from the GI tract. The usual route of administration is intermittent IV infusion or IM injection.

Aminoglycosides share common toxic effects, mainly nephrotoxicity and ototoxicity. Nephrotoxicity occurs in the proximal tubules and is manifested by increased serum creatinine and excretion of granular casts and protein. The nephrotoxicity is usually reversible if serum drug concentrations are monitored early in the course of therapy, prompt, appropriate adjustment of dosing is made, and renal function is followed closely. Ototoxicity causes both auditory and vestibular damage and is manifested by hearing loss (also dizziness, vertigo, ataxia, and tinnitus, which are difficult to assess in infancy). The ototoxicity may not be reversible. Audiometric testing may detect high-frequency hearing loss before clinical hearing loss is evident.

Aminoglycosides are eliminated unchanged in the urine. Kidney impairment will decrease elimination and cause accumulation of the drug with an increased potential for nephrotoxicity and ototoxicity.

Serum drug concentrations should be monitored early in the course of therapy and repeated at least once if the course of therapy is greater than 10 days. Initial peak and trough serum concentrations are typically sampled around the third dose (around the second dose if the dosing interval is q 24 hours). Trough serum concentrations should be drawn about 15 minutes before the dose. Peak serum concentrations should be drawn 1 hour after completion of a 30 minute IV infusion.

Ideally, gentamicin is used for empiric or proven Gram-negative coverage, while the other aminoglycosides are held in reserve for use against resistant strains of normally susceptible organisms.

The recommendations for the initial dosing of the aminoglycosides and of vancomycin are the result of our clinical observations and careful pharmacokinetic monitoring. While our recommendations differ from those of other authors, these guidelines provide safe, effective therapy. The built-in margin of safety is important if the ability to closely follow serum concentrations is limited or nonexistent.

Amikacin

Brand Names

Amikin

Forms

Injection 50 mg/ml in 2 ml vials; 250 mg/ml in 2 and 4 ml vials.

Uses

Aminoglycoside. Treatment of infections caused by susceptible Gram-negative bacteria: *Acinetobacter*, *Escherichia coli*, *Proteus mirabilis*, *Pseudomonas*, *Klebsiella*, *Enterobacter*, and *Serratia*. Treatment of susceptible Gram-positive bacteria: *Staphylococcus aureus* and *Staphylococcus epidermidis*.

Dose

Preterm infants <1000 gm	10 mg/kg/dose IV, IM q 24 hours
Preterm infants ≥1000 gm	10 mg/kg/dose IV, IM q 18 hours
Term infants	10 mg/kg/dose IV, IM q 18 hours

>1 month of age, the dosing intervals may be decreased by 6 hours.
>2 months of age, the dose should be decreased to 7.5 mg/kg/dose.

Pharmacokinetics

Bactericidal. Absorbed over 1 hour after IM administration. Distributes widely throughout the body, including soft tissues, heart, lung, and bone, and is also present in bile, sputum, and bronchial secretions. Penetration into CSF probably not sufficient to treat meningitis. Half-life is 3–9 hours and is related to urine output, glomerular filtration, and postnatal age. Eliminated unchanged in the urine. Immature or "asphyxiated" kidneys may decrease drug elimination. Therapeutic serum concentrations: Peak 20–30 mcg/ml.

Trough 8–10 mcg/ml.

Cautions

Expect drug accumulation with serum creatinine levels ≥0.8 mg/dl. The most common side effects include nephrotoxicity and ototoxicity. The nephrotoxicity may be reversible if the drug is discontinued or dose is adjusted promptly. The ototoxicity may be irreversible. (See "AMINOGLYCOSIDES," general statement.) Vomiting, leukopenia, thrombocytopenia, and hypersensitivity reactions with rash, fever, and eosinophilia are rare.

Use may result in overgrowth of nonsusceptible organisms including fungi.

Use with caution in infants with renal impairment or decreased urine output (<1–2 ml/kg/hr). Contraindicated in anuric infants except as a single dose, ONLY.

Solution Compatibility

D5W, D10W, 0.9% NaCl.

Additive Compatibility

Calcium gluconate, clindamycin, dexamethasone, potassium chloride, vancomycin.

Anti-Infectives

Additive Incompatibility

Aminophylline, amphotericin B, cephalosporins, heparin, penicillins, phenytoin.

Drug Interactions

Amphotericin B: increased risk of nephrotoxicity.
Cephalosporins: nephrotoxicity of both drugs may be increased.
Furosemide: increased risk of ototoxicity with possible severe permanent hearing loss.
Indomethacin: decreased amikacin elimination for 24–48 hours after last indomethacin dose.
Penicillins: antimicrobial effectiveness of aminoglycosides may be decreased by physiochemical inactivation if both drugs are administered at the same time.
Skeletal muscle relaxants (atracurium, pancuronium, succinylcholine, vecuronium): neuromuscular blocking effects of depolarizing and nondepolarizing muscle relaxants may be increased. Prolonged respiratory depression with extended periods of apnea may occur.
Vancomycin: increased risk of ototoxicity.

Nursing Considerations

- Obtain culture and sensitivity studies prior to initiation of therapy.
- CAREFUL attention to dose scheduling when q 18 hour interval is used.
- Infuse slowly IV over 30 minutes.
- Monitor kidney function (especially serum creatinine) and urine output.

- Maintain adequate urine output (≥2 ml/kg/hr).
- Question administration of dose in infants with inadequate urine output.
- Sample initial serum concentrations around the third dose (around the second dose if the dosing interval is q 24 hours) and then as indicated by changes in kidney function or changes in dosing.
  - trough: obtain blood 15 minutes before the dose.
  - peak: obtain blood 1 hour after completion of a 30 minute IV infusion (a true peak serum concentration is slightly higher than this value).
- Hold penicillin or cephalosporin doses for 2 hours before amikacin concentrations are drawn. Penicillins and cephalosporins degrade amikacin in vitro, and their presence in the serum sample may cause a falsely low amikacin concentration.
- Obtain audiometric testing (brainstem auditory evoked responses) prior to discharge.

Gentamicin

Brand Names

Garamycin, various

Forms

Injection 10 mg/ml and 40 mg/ml in 2 ml vials (contains preservatives).
2 mg/ml in 2 ml vials (nonpreserved) for intrathecal use.

Uses

Aminoglycoside. Treatment of infections caused by susceptible Gram-negative bacteria: *Escherichia coli,*

Klebsiella, and *Pseudomonas*. Treatment of susceptible Gram-positive bacteria: *Staphylococcus aureus* and *Staphylococcus epidermidis*.

Dose

Preterm infants <1000 gm	2.5 mg/kg/dose IV, IM q 24 hours.
Preterm infants ≥1000 gm	2.5 mg/kg/dose IV, IM q 18 hours.
Term infants	3 mg/kg/dose IV, IM q 18 hours.

>1 month of age, the dosing intervals may be decreased by 6 hours.

Pharmacokinetics

Bactericidal. Absorbed over 1 hour after IM administration. Distributes widely throughout the body, including soft tissues, heart, lung, and bone, and is also present in bile, sputum, and bronchial secretions. Penetration into CSF is negligible. Half-life is 3–6 hours (to 16 hours in the preterm infant) and is related to urine output, glomerular filtration, and postnatal age. Eliminated unchanged in urine. Immature or "asphyxiated" kidneys may decrease drug elimination. Therapeutic serum concentrations: Peak 5–8 mcg/ml
Trough <2 mcg/ml

Cautions

Expect drug accumulation with serum creatinine levels ≥0.8 mg/dl. The most common side effects include nephrotoxicity and ototoxicity. The nephrotoxicity may be reversible if the drug is discontinued or dose is adjusted promptly. The ototoxicity may be irreversible. See "AMINOGLYCOSIDES," general statement. Vomiting, leukopenia, thrombocytopenia, and hypersensitivity reactions with rash, fever, and eosinophilia are rare.

Use may result in overgrowth of nonsusceptible organisms including fungi.

Use with caution in infants with renal impairment or decreased urine output (<1–2 ml/kg/hr). Contraindicated in anuric infants except as a single dose, ONLY.

Solution Compatibility

D5W, D10W, 0.9% NaCl, TPN (without heparin).

Additive Compatibility

Cimetidine, clindamycin, metronidazole.

Additive Incompatibility

Cephalosporins, dopamine, furosemide, heparin, penicillins.

Drug Interactions

Amphotericin B: increased risk of nephrotoxicity.
Cephalosporins: nephrotoxicity of both drugs may be increased.
Furosemide: increased risk of ototoxicity with possible severe permanent hearing loss.
Indomethacin: decreased gentamicin elimination for 24–48 hours after last indomethacin dose.
Penicillins: antimicrobial effectiveness of aminoglycosides may be decreased by physiochemical

inactivation if both drugs are administered at the same time.

Skeletal muscle relaxants (atracurium, pancuronium, succinylcholine, vecuronium): neuromuscular blocking effects of depolarizing and nondepolarizing muscle relaxants may be increased. Prolonged respiratory depression with extended periods of apnea may occur.

Vancomycin: increased risk of ototoxicity.

Nursing Considerations

- Obtain culture and sensitivity studies prior to initiation of therapy.
- CAREFUL attention to dose scheduling when q 18 hour interval is used.
- Infuse slowly IV over 30 minutes.
- Monitor kidney function (especially serum creatinine) and urine output.
- Maintain adequate urine output (≥ 2 ml/kg/hr).
- Question administration of dose in infants with inadequate urine output.
- Sample initial serum concentrations around the third dose (around the second dose if the dosing interval is q 24 hours) and then as indicated by changes in kidney function or changes in dosing.
  - trough: obtain blood 15 minutes before the dose.
  - peak: obtain blood 1 hour after completion of a 30 minute IV infusion (a true peak serum concentration is slightly higher than this value).
- Hold penicillin or cephalosporin doses for 2 hours before gentamicin concentrations are drawn. Penicillins and cephalosporins degrade gentamicin in

vitro, and their presence in the serum sample may
cause a falsely low gentamicin concentration.
• Obtain audiometric testing (brainstem auditory
evoked responses) prior to discharge.

Tobramycin

Brand Names

Nebicin, various

Forms

Injection 10 mg/ml and 40 mg/ml in 2 ml vials.

Uses

Aminoglycoside. Treatment of infections caused by
susceptible Gram-negative bacteria: *Escherichia coli,
Klebsiella*, and *Pseudomonas*. Treatment of susceptible Gram-positive bacteria: *Staphylococcus aureus*
and *Staphylococcus epidermidis*.

Dose

Preterm infants <1000 gm	2.5 mg/kg/dose IV, IM q 24 hours
Preterm infants ≥1000 gm	2.5 mg/kg/dose IV, IM q 18 hours
Term infants	3 mg/kg/dose IV, IM q 18 hours

>1 month of age, the dosing intervals may be
decreased by 6 hours.

Pharmacokinetics

Bactericidal. Absorbed over 1 hour after IM administration. Distributes widely throughout the body,

including soft tissues, heart, lung, and bone, and is also present in bile, sputum, and bronchial secretions. Penetration into CSF is negligible. Half-life is 3–4.5 hours in the term infant (to 17 hours in the preterm infant) and is related to urine output, glomerular filtration, and postnatal age. Eliminated unchanged in the urine. Immature or "asphyxiated" kidneys may decrease drug elimination.

Therapeutic serum concentrations: Peak 5–8 mcg/ml.
Trough <2 mcg/ml.

Cautions

Expect drug accumulation with serum creatinine levels ≥0.8 mg/dl. The most common side effects include nephrotoxicity and ototoxicity. The nephrotoxicity may be reversible if the drug is discontinued or dose is adjusted promptly. The ototoxicity may be irreversible. (See "AMINOGLYCOSIDES," general statement.) Vomiting, leukopenia, thrombocytopenia, and hypersensitivity reactions with rash, fever, and eosinophilia are rare.

Use may result in overgrowth of nonsusceptible organisms including fungi.

Use with caution in infants with renal impairment or decreased urine output (<1–2 ml/kg/hr). Contraindicated in anuric infants except as a single dose, ONLY.

Solution Compatibility

D5W, D10W, 0.9% NaCl, TPN (without heparin).

Additive Compatibility

Furosemide, metronidazole.

Additive Incompatibility

Cephalosporins, heparin, penicillins.

Drug Interactions

Amphotericin B: increased risk of nephrotoxicity.
Cephalosporins: nephrotoxicity of both drugs may be increased.
Furosemide: increased risk of ototoxicity with possible severe permanent hearing loss.
Indomethacin: decreased tobramycin elimination for 24–48 hours after last indomethacin dose.
Penicillins: antimicrobial effectiveness of aminoglycosides may be decreased by physiochemical inactivation if both drugs are administered at the same time.
Skeletal muscle relaxants (atracurium, pancuronium, succinylcholine, vecuronium): neuromuscular blocking effects of depolarizing and nondepolarizing muscle relaxants may be increased. Prolonged respiratory depression with extended periods of apnea may occur.
Vancomycin: increased risk of ototoxicity.

Nursing Considerations

- Obtain culture and sensitivity studies prior to initiation of therapy.
- CAREFUL attention to dose scheduling when q 18 hour interval is used.
- Infuse slowly IV over 30 minutes.

- Monitor kidney function (especially serum creatinine) and urine output.
- Maintain adequate urine output (≥2 ml/kg/hr).
- Question administration of dose in infants with inadequate urine output.
- Sample initial serum concentrations around the third dose (around the second dose if the dosing interval is q 24 hours) and then as indicated by changes in kidney function or changes in dosing.
  - trough: obtain blood 15 minutes before the dose.
  - peak: obtain blood 1 hour after completion of a 30 minute IV infusion (a true peak concentration is slightly higher than this value).
- Hold penicillin or cephalosporin doses for 2 hours before tobramycin concentrations are drawn. Penicillins and cephalosporins degrade tobramycin in vitro, and their presence in the serum sample may cause a falsely low tobramycin concentration.
- Obtain audiometric testing (brainstem auditory evoked responses) prior to discharge.

CEPHALOSPORINS

Cefazolin

Brand Names

Ancef, Kefzol, various

Forms

Injection 250 mg, 500 mg, 1 gram vials (for reconstitution).

Uses

First-generation cephalosporin: active against non-methicillin-resistant *Staphylococcus*, susceptible strains of *Streptococcus, Klebsiella*, and *Escherichia coli*.
Prophylaxis prior to cardiothoracic surgery.

Dose

20 mg/kg/dose IV, IM q 8–12 hours.
Cardiothoracic surgery prophylaxis: 1 dose just prior to surgery followed by a 48-hour postoperative course of drug.
Eliminate 1 dose per day in infants with moderate to severe kidney impairment.

Pharmacokinetics

Bactericidal. Well absorbed after IM administration. Half-life is 3–4.5 hours. Penetration into CSF is negligible. Eliminated unchanged in the urine. Severe kidney impairment decreases drug clearance. Highly plasma protein bound.

Cautions

Hypersensitivity can cause rash and fever. Mild, reversible neutropenia and hypoprothrombinemia and nephrotoxicity (with increased BUN and creatinine) are rare. Can cause increase in SGOT, SGPT, and false-positive Coombs test (direct and indirect). Intramuscular route can cause pain, induration, and sterile abscess at injection site.

Prolonged use may result in overgrowth of nonsusceptible organisms, especially *Enterobacter, Pseudomonas*, enterococci, or *Candida*.

Use with caution in infants with kidney dysfunction or known hypersensitivity to penicillins.

Solution Compatibility

D5W, D10W, 0.45% NaCl, 0.9% NaCl, TPN.

Additive Incompatibility

Amikacin, calcium gluconate, gentamicin, tobramycin, and strongly alkaline solutions.

Drug Interactions

Aminoglycosides (amikacin, gentamicin, tobramycin): nephrotoxicity of both drugs may be increased.

Nursing Considerations

- Obtain culture and sensitivity studies prior to initiation of therapy.
- Infuse slowly IV over 15–30 minutes.
- Use IM route only in infants without IV access.
- Observe for rash.
- Monitor infant's temperature.
- Monitor kidney function and urine output.
- Protect reconstituted drug from light.
- Sodium content: 2 mEq/gm.
- Osmolaltity (Kefzol 225 mg/ml):636 mOsm/kg H_2O (FP).

Cefotaxime

Brand Name

Claforan

Forms

Injection 500 mg, 1 gram, 2 gram vials (for reconstitution) IV use only.

Uses

Third-generation cephalosporin: active against gram-negative bacteria *Escherichia coli, Haemophilus influenzae, Klebsiella pneumoniae, Neisseria gonnorrhea, Proteus mirabilis,* and *Serratia.*

Dose

50 mg/kg/dose IV q 12 hours in infants ≤1 week of age.
50 mg/kg/dose IV q 8 hours in infants >1 week of age.
Eliminate 1 dose per day in infants with severe kidney impairment.

Pharmacokinetics

Bactericidal. Distributes widely into most body fluids and tissues. Half-life is 2–6 hours. Metabolized in the liver primarily to an active metabolite (desacetylcefotaxime) and some inactive metabolites which are eliminated in the urine. With inflamed meninges, CSF concentration is 30–60% of the serum concentration. Moderately plasma protein bound.

Cautions

Hypersensitivity can cause rash and fever. Transient neutropenia, granulocytopenia and leukopenia, and rarely nephrotoxicity (with increased BUN and creatinine) can occur. Can cause phlebitis at IV injection site.

Prolonged use may result in overgrowth of nonsusceptible organisms, especially *Enterobacter, Pseudomonas*, enterococci, or *Candida*.

Use with caution in infants with kidney dysfunction or known hypersensitivity to penicillins.

Solution Compatibility

D5W, D10W, 0.9% NaCl, TPN.

Additive Incompatibility

Amikacin, aminophylline, gentamicin, sodium bicarbonate, tobramycin.

Drug Interactions

Aminoglycosides (amikacin, gentamicin, tobramycin): nephrotoxicity of both drugs may be increased.

Nursing Considerations

- Obtain culture and sensitivity studies prior to initiation of therapy.
- Infuse slowly IV push over 15 minutes.
- Observe for rash.
- Monitor infant's temperature.
- Monitor kidney function and urine output.
- Monitor CBC with differential weekly.
- Protect from light and heat.
- Sodium content: 2.2 mEq/gm.

Ceftazidime

Brand Names

Fortaz, Tazidime

Forms

Injection 500 mg, 1 gram, 2 gram vials (for reconstitution).

Uses

Third-generation cephalosporin: active against susceptible strains of *Pseudomonas* and also active against *E. coli, H. influenzae, Klebsiella, Neisseria,* and *Serratia.*

Dose

30–50 mg/kg/dose IV q 8–12 hours.
Administer q 24 hours in infants with severe kidney impairment.

Pharmacokinetics

Bactericidal. Distributes widely into many body tissues, including CSF. Eliminated unchanged in the urine. Severe kidney impairment decreases drug clearance.

Cautions

Hypersensitivity can cause rash, fever, and eosinophilia. Mild, reversible neutropenia and nephrotoxicity (with increased BUN and creatinine) are rare.

Prolonged use may result in overgrowth of nonsusceptible organisms, especially *Enterobacter, Pseudomonas,* enterococci, or *Candida.*

Use with caution in infants with kidney dysfunction or known hypersensitivity to penicillins.

Solution Compatibility

Dextrose-saline combinations, D5W, D10W, 0.45% NaCl, 0.9% NaCl.

Additive Incompatibility

Amikacin, gentamicin, tobramycin, and strongly alkaline solutions.

Drug Interactions

Aminoglycosides (amikacin, gentamicin, tobramycin): nephrotoxicity of both drugs may be increased.

Nursing Considerations

- Obtain culture and sensitivity studies prior to initiation of therapy.
- Reconstitute just prior to administration. Reconstitution of drug produces carbon dioxide and causes pressure within the vial. Precaution should be taken to vent the carbon dioxide gas.
- Infuse slowly IV push over 15 minutes.
- Observe for rash.
- Monitor infant's temperature.
- Monitor kidney function and urine output.
- Protect from light.
- Sodium content: 2.3 mEq/gm.

Ceftriaxone

Brand Name

Rocephin

Forms

Injection 250 mg, 500 mg, 1 gram, 2 gram vials.

Uses

Third-generation cephalosporin: excellent activity against the most common pathogens of childhood: *Haemophilus influenzae, Neisseria meningitidis*, and *Streptococcus pneumoniae*. Also excellent activity against *Escherichia coli, Klebsiella pneumoniae, Neisseria gonorrhea, Proteus mirabilis*, and *Serratia*.

Dose

25 mg/kg/dose IV, IM q 12 hours.
Meningitis: 50 mg/kg/dose IV, IM q 12 hours.
Administer q 24 hours in infants with severe liver and kidney impairment.
Gonococcal prophylaxis: 25–50 mg/kg/dose IM once.
Gonococcal ophthalmia treatment: 25–50 mg IM q 24 hours for 7 days.

Pharmacokinetics

Bactericidal. Distributes widely in many body fluids and tissues. Half-life is 4–8 hours, up to 16 hours in the preterm infant. Cerebrospinal fluid concentration is 10% of serum concentration, sufficient to treat meningitis. Eliminated unchanged primarily by the kidneys in urine and also by the liver in bile. Highly plasma protein bound.

Cautions

Hypersensitivity can cause rash, fever, and eosinophilia. Rarely, anemia, leukopenia, neutropenia, thrombocytopenia, nephrotoxicity (with increased BUN and creatinine), and increased SGOT, SGPT, and bilirubin can occur. Can cause phlebitis at IV injection site and pain and tenderness at IM injection site. May displace bilirubin from albumin binding sites.

Prolonged use may result in overgrowth of nonsusceptible organisms, especially *Enterobacter, Pseudomonas*, enterococci, or *Candida*.

Use with caution in infants with liver and/or kidney dysfunction or known hypersensitivity to penicillins.

Solution Compatibility

D5W, D10W, 0.9% NaCl, TPN.

Additive Compatibility

Compatible with lidocaine 1% only. Do NOT mix with other drugs.

Drug Interactions

Aminoglycosides (amikacin, gentamicin, tobramycin): nephrotoxicity of both drugs may be increased.

Nursing Considerations

- Obtain culture and sensitivity studies prior to initiation of therapy.
- Infuse slowly IV push over 15 minutes.
- Observe for rash.
- Monitor infant's temperature.
- Monitor liver and kidney function.
- Monitor CBC with differential and platelet count weekly.
- Intramuscular route very painful. Manufacturer recommends mixing IM dose with lidocaine 1% WITHOUT epinephrine.
- Sodium content: 3.6 mEq/gm.

PENICILLINS

Ampicillin

Brand Names

Omnipen, Polycillin, Totacillin, various

Forms

Injection 125 mg, 250 mg, 500 mg, 1 gram, 2 gram vials (for reconstitution).
Oral suspension 125 mg/5 ml, 250 mg/5 ml, in 100 ml and 200 ml bottles.

Uses

Treatment of infections caused by susceptible strains of Streptococci groups A, B, C, and G, *Streptococcus pneumoniae, Listeria monocytogenes, Haemophilus influenzae*, non-penicillinase-producing strains of *Neisseria gonorrhea* and *Neisseria meningitidis*, and other susceptible organisms including *Streptococcus faecalis, Clostridium, Escherichia coli, Salmonella*, and *Shigella*.

Dose

50–100 mg/kg/dose IV, IM q 12 hours in infants ≤1 week of age.
Meningitis: 200 mg/kg/day IV q 12 hours in infants ≤ 1 week of age.
Administer q 8 hours in infants >1 week of age, q 6 hours >1 month of age.
50–100 mg/kg/day PO q 6 hours.

Anti-Infectives

Pharmacokinetics

Bactericidal. Good absorption (30–55%) from the GI tract. Food will decrease extent and rate of absorption. Excellent absorption after IM administration. Sufficient CSF concentration (11–65% of serum concentration) after IV administration to treat meningitis. Drug concentrates in bile and urine. Half-life is about 4 hours and decreases with postnatal age to <2 hours at 30 days of life. Primarily eliminated unchanged in the urine.

Cautions

Hypersensitivity can cause urticarial and/or maculopapular rash, fever, anemia, eosinophilia, and rarely, anaphylaxis. Diarrhea (PO administration), interstitial nephritis (with hematuria), and rarely, bone marrow suppression (with anemia, leukopenia, neutropenia, thrombocytopenia, or rarely, agranulocytosis) can occur.

Use may result in overgrowth of nonsusceptible organisms including *Candida, Enterobacter, Klebsiella, E. coli, Aerobacter,* and *Pseudomonas.*

Use with caution in infants with kidney dysfunction or known hypersensitivity to cephalosporins or other penicillins.

Solution Compatibility

D5W, D10W, 0.9% NaCl, TPN if infusion is ≤30 minutes.

Additive Compatibility

Heparin.

Additive Incompatibility

Amikacin, dopamine, gentamicin, tobramycin, and strongly alkaline solutions.

Drug Interactions

Aminoglycosides (amikacin, gentamicin, tobramycin): antimicrobial effectiveness of aminoglycosides may be decreased by physiochemical inactivation if both drugs are administered at the same time.

Nursing Considerations

- Commonly used in combination with an aminoglycoside as initial treatment for suspected or confirmed bacterial infections.
- Obtain culture and sensitivity studies prior to initiation of therapy.
- Use reconstituted drug within an hour to avoid loss of potency.
- Infuse slowly IV push over 15–30 minutes.
- Use IM route only in infants without IV access.
- Shake suspension well before drawing up dose.
- Administer PO preparation 1 hour before or 2 hours after a feeding.
- Observe for rash.
- Monitor infant's temperature.
- Observe for evidence of thrush or candidal diaper rash.
- Monitor kidney function and urine output.
- Test urine for protein and blood.
- Monitor CBC and platelet count.
- Sodium content: 3 mEq/gm.
- Osmolality (Omnipen 125 mg/ml): 702 mOsm/kg

H_2O (FP).
(Polycillin 125 mg/ml): 675 mOsm/kg
H_2O (FP).

Methicillin

Brand Name

Staphcillin

Forms

Injection 1 gram vials (for reconstitution).

Uses

Semisynthetic, penicillinase-resistant penicillin. Used primarily for the treatment of infections caused by non-methicillin-resistant strains of *Staphylococcus aureus* and *Staphylococcus epidermidis*.

Dose

25 mg/kg/dose IV, IM q 8–12 hours in infants ≤1 week of age.
Meningitis: 50 mg/kg/dose IV q 8 hours in infants ≤1 week of age.
Administer q 6 hours in infants >1 week of age.

Pharmacokinetics

Bactericidal. Inactivated by acidic gastric secretions with PO administration; thus must be administered parentally. Rapidly and well absorbed after IM administration. Penetration into CSF is about 10% of concurrent serum concentration. Half-life is 1–3 hours. No appreciable metabolism. Primarily eliminated unchanged in the urine. Elimination increases with postnatal age.

Cautions

Hypersensitivity can cause urticarial rash, fever, anemia, eosinophilia, and rarely, anaphylaxis. Interstitial nephritis (with hematuria, proteinuria, and casts in the urine), and rarely, bone marrow suppression (with anemia, leukopenia, neutropenia, thrombocytopenia or rarely, agranulocytosis) and hepatotoxicity (with increased alkaline phosphatase, SGPT, SGOT, LDH) can occur. Incidence of interstitial nephritis is greater with methicillin than nafcillin or oxacillin, and the incidence of hepatotoxicity may be less than with oxacillin. Intravenous administration can cause phlebitis or thrombophlebitis. Intramuscular administration can cause pain and sterile abscess.

Prolonged use may result in overgrowth of nonsusceptible organisms including fungi or Gram-negative bacteria such as *Pseudomonas*.

Use with caution in infants with kidney dysfunction or known hypersensitivity to cephalosporins or other penicillins.

Solution Compatibility

D5W, D10W, 0.9% NaCl, TPN.

Additive Compatibility

Aminophylline, heparin.

Additive Incompatibility

Amikacin, gentamicin, morphine, sodium bicarbonate, tobramycin, vancomycin.

Anti-Infectives   **157**

Drug Interactions

Aminoglycosides (amikacin, gentamicin, tobramycin): antimicrobial effectiveness of aminoglycosides may be decreased by physiochemical inactivation if both drugs are administered at the same time.

Nursing Considerations

- Obtain culture and sensitivity studies prior to initiation of therapy.
- Infuse slowly IV push over 15–30 minutes.
- Use IM route only in infants without IV access.
- Observe for rash.
- Monitor temperature.
- Observe for thrush or candidal diaper rash.
- Monitor kidney function and urine output.
- Test urine for protein and blood.
- Monitor liver function.
- Monitor CBC and platelet count.
- Sodium content: 2.5 mEq/gm.

Nafcillin

Brand Names

Unipen, Nafcil

Forms

Injection 500 mg, 1 gram, 2 gram vials (for reconstitution).

Uses

Semisynthetic, penicillinase-resistant penicillin. Used primarily for the treatment of infections caused by non-methicillin-resistant strains of *Staphylococcus aureus* and *Staphylococcus epidermidis*.

Dose

20–25 mg/kg/dose IV, IM q 12 hours in infants ≤1 week of age.
Meningitis: 50 mg/kg/dose IV q 12 hours in infants ≤1 week of age.
Administer q 8 hours in infants >1 week of age.

Pharmacokinetics

Bactericidal. Poorly and erratically absorbed from the GI tract. Rapidly and well absorbed after IM administration. Penetration into CSF greater than that of methicillin and is sufficient to treat some CNS infections. Half-life is 3–4 hours. Metabolized to inactive metabolites and eliminated in the bile with some drug eliminated unchanged in the urine. Moderately plasma protein bound.

Cautions

Hypersensitivity can cause urticarial rash, fever, anemia, eosinophilia, and rarely, anaphylaxis. Interstitial nephritis (with hematuria, proteinuria, and casts in the urine), and rarely, bone marrow suppression (with anemia, leukopenia, neutropenia, thrombocytopenia, or rarely, agranulocytosis) and hepatotoxicity (with increased alkaline phosphatase, SGPT, SGOT, LDH) can occur. The incidence of hepatotoxicity may be less with nafcillin than with oxacillin. Intravenous administration can cause phlebitis or thrombophlebitis. Extravasation can cause tissue necrosis and sloughing. Intramuscular administration can cause pain and sterile abscess.

Prolonged use may result in overgrowth of nonsusceptible organisms including fungi or Gram-negative bacteria such as *Pseudomonas*.

Use with caution in infants with kidney dysfunction or known hypersensitivity to cephalosporins or other penicillins.

Solution Compatibility

D5W, D10W, 0.45% NaCl, 0.9% NaCl, TPN.

Additive Compatibility

Aminophylline, cimetidine, dexamethasone, heparin.

Additive Incompatibility

Amikacin, gentamicin, hydrocortisone, methylprednisolone, tobramycin.

Drug Interactions

Aminoglycosides (amikacin, gentamicin, tobramycin): antimicrobial effectiveness of aminoglycosides may be decreased by physiochemical inactivation if both drugs are administered at the same time.

Nursing Considerations

- Obtain culture and sensitivity studies prior to initiation of therapy.
- Infuse slowly IV push over 15–30 minutes.
- Observe IV site closely for extravasation. Treatment for extravasation: Hyaluronidase (Wydase) 150 unit vial reconstituted with 1 ml of NS. Infiltrate

throughout affected area as soon as possible. Use 25 gauge needle.

- Use IM route only in infants without IV access.
- Observe for rash.
- Monitor temperature.
- Observe for thrush or candidal diaper rash.
- Monitor kidney function and urine output.
- Monitor urine for protein and blood.
- Monitor liver function.
- Monitor CBC and platelet count.
- Sodium content: 2.9 mEq/gm.
- Osmolality (Unipen 250 mg/ml): 709 mOsm/kg H_2O (FP).

Penicillin G

Brand Name

Pfizerpen

Forms

Penicillin G potassium injection 500,000 unit, 1,000,000 unit vials (for reconstitution). Sodium salt also available.
Benzathine penicillin G 300,000 unit, 600,000 unit pre-loaded syringe.
Procaine penicillin G 300,000 unit, 500,000 unit, 600,000 unit syringe.

Uses

Treatment of infections caused by susceptible strains of Streptococci groups A, B, C, and G, *Streptococcus pneumoniae*, and non-penicillinase-producing strains of *Neisseria gonorrhea* and *Neisseria meningitidis*.

Treatment of congenital syphilis.

Dose

25,000–50,000 units/kg/dose IV, IM q 12 hours in infants ≤1 week of age.
Administer q 8 hours in infants >1 week of age.
Meningitis: 75,000–100,000 units/kg/dose IV q 8 hours ≤1 week of age.
Administer q 6 hours in infants >1 week of age.
Benzathine penicillin G 50,000 units/kg/dose IM. One dose for treatment of asymptomatic congenital syphilis.
Procaine penicillin G 50,000 units/kg/dose IM q 24 hours for 10 days for treatment of congenital syphilis without CNS involvement and for 14–21 days for congenital syphilis with CNS involvement.

Pharmacokinetics

Bactericidal. Gastric acidity destroys penicillin G, limiting usefulness of oral route. (Penicillin V is acid-stable and preferred for oral route.) Rapidly and well absorbed after IM administration. Widely distributed throughout the body, but concentrations in various tissues and fluids differ greatly. Cerebrospinal fluid concentration is ≤10% of serum concentration. Half-life is 1–2.5 hours. Primarily eliminated unchanged in the urine with <10% of drug metabolized. Moderately plasma protein bound.

Cautions

Hypersensitivity can cause rash, fever, anemia, eosinophilia, and anaphylaxis. Interstitial nephritis (with fever, hematuria, and proteinuria) and rarely, bone

marrow suppression (with transient neutropenia, leukopenia, and thrombocytopenia) and hepatotoxicity
(with increased SGOT and LDH) can occur. Drug
accumulation can cause drowsiness, hyperreflexia,
twitching, myoclonus, and seizures. Serious and
potentially fatal electrolyte disturbances, due to the
sodium and potassium content of drug, can occur.
Rapid IV infusion or overdosing can cause seizures
and rarely, cardiac arrhythmias and arrest.

Use may result in overgrowth of nonsusceptible
organisms, especially *Candida, Enterobacter,* or *Pseudomonas;* increased incidence with indwelling
catheters.

Use with caution in infants with kidney dysfunction
or known hypersensitivity to cephalosporins or other
penicillins.

Solution Compatibility

D5W, D10W, 0.9% NaCl, TPN.

Additive Compatibility

Cimetidine, clindamycin, heparin, morphine.

Additive Incompatibility

Amikacin, aminophylline, dopamine, gentamicin,
sodium bicarbonate, tobramycin, and strongly acidic
or alkaline solutions.

Drug Interactions

Aminoglycosides (amikacin, gentamicin, tobramycin):
antimicrobial effectiveness of aminoglycosides may be
decreased by physiochemical inactivation if both
drugs are administered at the same time.

Nursing Considerations

- Obtain culture and sensitivity studies prior to initiation of therapy.
- Infuse slowly IV over 15–30 minutes (penicillin G potassium or sodium).
- Use IM route ONLY for benzathine or procaine Penicillin G; IV administration can cause severe vascular damage.
- Observe for rash.
- Monitor infant's temperature.
- Observe for thrush or candidal diaper rash.
- Monitor serum electrolytes (especially potassium and sodium).
- Monitor kidney function and urine output.
- Monitor liver function.
- Monitor CBC and platelet count.
- Potassium content: 1.7 mEq/1 million units (potassium penicillin G). Sodium content: 2.0 mEq/1 million units (sodium penicillin G).
- Osmolality (Pfizerpen 250,000 units/ml): 776 mOsm/kg H_2O (FP).

Piperacillin

Brand Name

Pipercil

Forms

Injection 2 gram, 3 gram, 4 gram vials (for reconstitution).

Uses

Used primarily for the treatment of infections caused by susceptible strains of *Pseudomonas aeruginosa* and also *Klebsiella, Enterobacter, Escherichia coli*, and *Proteus*.

Dose

Preterm infants ≤1 week of age 50 mg/kg/dose IV, IM q 8 hours.
>1 week of age 50 mg/kg/dose IV, IM q 6 hours.
Term infants 50 mg/kg/dose IV, IM q 6 hours.

Pharmacokinetics

Bactericidal. Not appreciably absorbed from the GI tract. Good absorption after IM administration. Poor CSF penetration, though concentrations increase in the presence of inflamed meninges. Concentrates in bile and urine. Half-life is up to 3.5 hours in newborns less than 1 week old. Primarily eliminated unchanged in the urine, with 20–30% eliminated unchanged in the bile; <10% of drug is metabolized.

Cautions

Hypersensitivity can cause rash, fever, anemia, and eosinophilia. Interstitial nephritis (with hematuria), bone marrow suppression (with anemia, leukopenia, neutropenia, or thrombocytopenia), and a transient increase in liver enzymes (alkaline phosphatase, SGOT, SGPT, bilirubin) can occur. Intravenous administration can cause pain, erythema, phlebitis, and thrombophlebitis. Intramuscular administration can cause pain, erythema, and induration.

Use may result in overgrowth of nonsusceptible organisms including *Candida, Pseudomonas, Serratia,* or *Klebsiella;* increased incidence with indwelling catheters.

Use with caution in infants with kidney or liver dysfunction or known hypersensitivity to cephalosporins or other penicillins.

Solution Compatibility

D5W, D10W, 0.9% NaCl, TPN.

Additive Compatibility

Clindamycin, heparin, morphine.

Additive Incompatibility

Amikacin, gentamicin, tobramycin.

Drug Interactions

Aminoglycosides (amikacin, gentamicin, tobramycin): antimicrobial effectiveness of aminoglycosides may be decreased by physiochemical inactivation if both drugs are administered at the same time.

Nursing Considerations

- Obtain culture and sensitivity studies prior to initiation of the therapy.
- Infuse slowly IV over 15–30 minutes.
- Use IM route only in infants without IV access.
- May mix IM dose with lidocaine 1% WITHOUT epinephrine to decrease pain.
- Observe for rash.
- Monitor infant's temperature.

- Observe for thrush or candidal diaper rash.
- Monitor kidney function and urine output.
- Monitor urine for protein and blood.
- Monitor liver function.
- Monitor CBC and platelet count and observe for signs of bleeding.
- Sodium content: 1.8 mEq/gm.

SULFONAMIDES

Sulfamethoxazole/Trimethoprim (SMX-TMP, Co-trimoxazole)

Brand Names

Bactrim, Septra, various

Forms

Injection trimethoprim 16 mg and sulfamethoxazole 80 mg/ml.
Oral suspension trimethoprim 8 mg and sulfamethoxazole 40 mg/ml (fixed combination—SMX:TMP is 5:1 ratio).

Uses

Treatment of urinary tract infections caused by many Gram-positive and Gram-negative bacteria, including *Escherichia coli, Proteus, Klebsiella*, and *Enterobacter*.
Treatment of otitis media caused by ampicillin-resistant *Haemophilus influenzae* or in penicillin-allergic infants.

Anti-Infectives

Dose

0.125 ml/kg/day IV q 12 hours.
0.25 ml/kg/day PO q 12 hours.
(trimethoprim 2 mg/kg/day and sulfamethoxazole 10 mg/kg/day.)
Decrease dose in infants with kidney dysfunction.
Requires good urine output (>2 ml/kg/hr).

Pharmacokinetics

Bactericidal (sulfamethoxazole is bacteriostatic and trimethoprim is bactericidal). Rapidly absorbed from the GI tract. Widely distributed throughout the body concentrating in the urine and the middle ear. Drug concentration in CSF is 40–50% serum concentration in the presence of inflamed meninges. Metabolized in the liver and excreted in the urine as metabolites and unchanged drug. Sulfamethoxazole is a weaker displacer of bilirubin than other sulfonamides.

Cautions

Can cause vomiting and poor feeding with oral route. Can cause hypersensitivity reactions with rash and fever. Anemia, neutropenia, thrombocytopenia, and severe skin reactions to sulfonamides (erythematous, maculopapular rashes, exfoliative dermatitis, and Stevens-Johnson syndrome) rarely occur. Toxic effects are reversible if drug is discontinued. Thrombophlebitis can occur with IV use. Sulfonamides may crystallize in kidneys with inadequate urine output.

Solution Compatibility

D5W (stable for 4 hours).

Additive Compatibility

Do NOT mix with other drugs.

Drug Interactions

Folic acid: trimethoprim may alter the metabolism of folic acid.

Phenytoin: effects of phenytoin may be increased with possible elevated plasma levels and toxicity.

Nursing Considerations

- Obtain culture and sensitivity studies prior to initiation of therapy.
- Intravenous form requires large volumes of D5W to keep drug in solution: 25 ml D5W for each ml sulfamethoxazole/trimethoprim.
- Infuse slowly IV over 1 hour.
- Observe IV site for signs of thrombophlebitis.
- Shake suspension well before drawing up dose.
- Administer PO preparation with feeding.
- Monitor kidney function and urine output.
- Maintain adequate urine output (>2 ml/kg/hour).
- Monitor CBC, differential, platelets.
- Discontinue drug at first sign of rash.
- Protect from light.

OTHER ANTIBIOTICS

Clindamycin

Brand Names

Cleocin, various

Forms

Injection 150 mg/ml in 2 ml, 4 ml, and 6 ml vials (contains benzyl alcohol).
Oral solution from granules 75 mg/5 ml (contains paraben preservatives).

Use

Treatment of infections caused by susceptible strains of anaerobic bacteria: *Actinomyces, Bacteroides, Peptococcus, Peptostreptococcus, Clostridium perfringens, Clostridium tetani,* and *Corynebacterium diphtheria.*
Inactive against *Clostridium difficile.*

Dose

≤1 month of age 5 mg/kg/dose IV, PO q 8 hours (severe infections q 6 hours).
>1 month of age 10 mg/kg/dose IV, PO q 8 hours (severe infections q 6 hours).

Pharmacokinetics

Bacteriostatic or bactericidal. Rapidly and completely absorbed after PO administration. Distributes widely throughout body tissues and fluids, including abscesses. Poor CSF penetration. Clindamycin is a "pro-drug" that is hydrolyzed to its free, active form in the GI tract, after PO administration, and in the plasma, after IV administration. Half-life is 3.5–4.7 hours in the term infant and 8.5–11 hours in the preterm infant. Metabolized in the liver to bioactive and inactive metabolites and excreted in the bile, feces, and urine with small amounts of unchanged drug. Highly plasma protein bound.

Cautions

Most serious side effect is pseudomembranous colitis characterized by fever, severe diarrhea, abdominal cramps, and blood and mucus in the stools. This syndrome is due to the production of an endotoxin by clindamycin-resistant strains of *Clostridium difficile* and can be fatal. Drug should be discontinued if signs of pseudomembranous colitis occur, and treatment with oral vancomycin 15 mg/kg/day divided into 3 or 4 doses for 7–10 days should be considered.

Can also cause vomiting, "simple" diarrhea, anorexia, rash, fever, transient neutropenia, leukopenia, eosinophilia, and thrombocytopenia, a transient increase in serum bilirubin, SGOT, and alkaline phosphatase, and hypotension and cardiopulmonary arrest (with rapid IV infusion). Pain, swelling, erythema, and thrombophlebitis at injection site can occur.

Use may result in overgrowth of nonsusceptible organisms, particularly fungi.

Use with caution in infants with liver dysfunction or GI disease.

Solution Compatibility

D5W, D10W, 0.9% NaCl, TPN.

Additive Compatibility

Amikacin, cimetidine, gentamicin, heparin, penicillin G, potassium chloride, sodium bicarbonate.

Additive Incompatibility

Aminophylline, ampicillin, calcium gluconate.

Drug Interactions

Skeletal muscle relaxants (atracurium, pancuronium, vecuronium): neuromuscular blocking effect of nonde-polarizing muscle relaxants may be increased. Prolonged respiratory depression with extended periods of apnea may occur.

Nursing Considerations

- Obtain culture and sensitivity studies prior to initia-tion of therapy.
- Infuse slowly IV over 30 minutes.
- Administer PO preparation with feeding to decrease GI irritation.
- Observe infant for diarrhea and check stools for blood (occult and gross) and mucus. Measure stool output.
- Monitor HR and rhythm, RR, and BP during infusion.
- Monitor liver and kidney function.
- Monitor CBC and platelet count.
- Observe for rash.
- Monitor infant's temperature.
- Do NOT refrigerate oral solution.
- Osmolality (Cleocin IV 150 mg/ml): 835 mOsm/kg H_2O (FP).
        (Cleocin PO 75 mg/5 ml): 1310 mOsm/kg H_2O (FP).

Erythromycin

Brand Names

Ilosone, Ilotycin, E.E.S., various

Forms

Injection 250 mg, 500 mg, 1 gram vials (for reconstitution).
Various oral suspensions available (contain paraben preservatives).
Various salt forms available: ethylsuccinate (PO), estolate (PO), lactobionate (IV), gluceptate (IV), and stearate (PO).
Ophthalmic ointment 0.5%.

Uses

Treatment of infections caused by susceptible strains of *Staphylococcus, Streptococcus, Bacillus anthracis, Clostridium, Corynebacterium, Bordatella*, and some strains of *Chlamydia, Rickettsia, Mycoplasma pneumoniae*, and *Ureaplasma urealyticum*.
Prevention of ophthalmia neonatorum.

Dose

Oral 20 mg/kg/dose PO q 12 hours.
Prevention of ophthalmia neonatorum: place a "ribbon" of 0.5% ointment in each lower conjunctival sac soon after birth.

Pharmacokinetics

Bacteriostatic or bactericidal. Well absorbed in the duodenum after PO administration. Distributes widely throughout body tissues and fluids, except CSF. Half-life of the ethylsuccinate salt is 2.5 hours and the half-life of the estolate salt is 6 hours. Some metabolism to inactive metabolites. Eliminated mainly as active drug in the bile with very small amounts eliminated in the urine.

Cautions

Abdominal pain (which can be quite severe), vomiting, and diarrhea are common. Hypersensitivity with rash, skin eruptions, and rarely, anaphylaxis can occur. Rarely hepatotoxicity with cholestatic hepatitis (with increased bilirubin and jaundice) may occur with use of the estolate or ethylsuccinate salts. Symptoms disappear over 1–2 weeks after the drug is discontinued, and liver function tests return to normal over 1–2 months. May falsely elevate urinary catecholamines (17-hydroxycortocosteroids and 17-ketosteroids).

Prolonged or repeated use may result in overgrowth of nonsusceptible bacteria or fungi.

Use with caution in infants with liver dysfunction.

Drug Interactions

Aminophylline/theophylline: effects of theophylline may be increased with possible elevated plasma levels and toxicity. Effectiveness of erythromycin may be decreased.
Corticosteroids: effects of certain corticosteriods may be increased.
Digoxin: increased digoxin serum levels with increased therapeutic and toxic effects. Effect of interaction may occur up to several months after discontinuation of erythromycin.

Nursing Considerations

- Obtain culture and sensitivity studies prior to initiation of therapy.
- Shake oral suspension well before drawing up dose.

- Administer on an empty stomach (presence of food can decrease absorption); however, administration with feeding may decrease GI irritation.
- Observe infant for vomiting, diarrhea, and signs of abdominal pain (irritability, drawing up of legs, tensing of abdomen with palpation).
- Monitor liver function and observe for jaundice.
- Observe for rash.
- Administer ophthalmic ointment to the lower conjunctival sac of open eye; then gently close eye and manipulate to ensure distribution of ointment.

NOTE Injectable form of drug is available. Severe vein irritation occurs with IV route. Injectable form must be diluted to a final concentration of 1 mg/ml. Dextrose 5% is the recommended diluent. The addition of sodium bicarbonate is necessary to keep erythromycin stable in solution. Infants may not be able to tolerate the volume of solution or the amount of sodium bicarbonate required to deliver the drug. Do NOT administer IM.

Metronidazole

Brand Names

Flagyl RTU (ready to use), various

Forms

Injection 5 mg/ml in normal saline for IV use (stabilized with sodium bicarbonate).
Tablets 250 mg, 500 mg (can be made into oral suspension).

Anti-Infectives   **175**

Uses

Treatment of infections caused by anaerobic bacteria, including *Bacteroides fragilis, Clostridium,* and *Actinomyces.*

Dose

Loading dose: 15 mg/kg IV.
Maintenance: 7.5 mg/kg/dose IV, PO q 12 hours.
                Start maintenance 12 hours after
                loading dose.
Increase dosing interval in infants with severe liver impairment.

Pharmacokinetics

Bactericidal, amebicidal, and trichomonacidal. Well absorbed from the GI tract. Drug distributes throughout the body. Half-life ranges from 25–75 hours. Metabolized in the liver to inactive metabolites and is excreted in the urine.

Cautions

Animal studies raise the concern of potential carcinogenicity, but adult human retrospective studies fail to show an increased incidence of cancer. Clindamycin is an alternative drug choice. Can cause abdominal discomfort, vomiting, and diarrhea with the oral route. May color urine a deep red-brown. Can cause erythematous rash, neutropenia, and, rarely, possible pseudomembranous colitis. Thrombophlebitis can occur with IV route. Can produce falsely low SGOT and SGPT.

Use may result in overgrowth of *Candida.*

Use with caution in preterm infants and infants with severe liver dysfunction.

Solution Compatibility

D5W, 0.9% NaCl, lactated Ringer's.

Additive Compatibility

Do NOT mix with other drugs.

Drug Interactions

Phenobarbital: increases metabolism of metronidazole resulting in decreased effectiveness.
Ethyl alcohol (in elixirs, KCl): causes disulfiram-like reaction (vomiting, abdominal cramps, sweating).

Nursing Considerations

- Obtain culture and sensitivity studies prior to initiation of therapy.
- Infuse slowly IV over 1 hour.
- Observe IV site for signs of thrombophlebitis.
- Shake suspension well before drawing up dose.
- Administer PO preparation with feeding.
- Observe for thrush and/or candidal diaper rash.
- Monitor liver function.
- Refrigerate oral suspension.
- Do NOT refrigerate IV preparation, or precipitation will occur.
- Protect from light.
- Sodium content (RTU form): 28 mEq/gram.

Vancomycin

Brand Names

Vancocin, various

Forms

Injection 500 mg vial (for reconstitution).

Uses

Treatment of life-threatening infections caused by methicillin-resistant strains of *Staphylococcus epidermidis* and *Staphylococcus aureus*.
Used orally for the treatment of colitis associated with *Clostridium difficile*.

Dose

Starting IV	Postnatal age	
doses:	0–30 days	30–60 days
Preterm infants <1000 gm	15 mg/kg/dose q 24 hours.	15 mg/kg/dose q 18 hours.
Preterm infants ≥1000 gm	15 mg/kg/dose q 18 hours.	15 mg/kg/dose q 12 hours.
Term infants	15 mg/kg/dose q 12 hours.	15 mg/kg/dose q 8 hours.

Infants greater than 60 days postnatal age: 10 mg/kg/dose IV q 6 hours.
Oral dose for colitis associated with *Clostridium difficile*: 15 mg/kg/day PO divided into 3–4 doses. Treat for 7–10 days.

Pharmacokinetics

Bactericidal. Widely distributed throughout the body, including CSF in the presence of inflamed meninges. Half-life ranges from 6–10 hours. Primarily eliminated unchanged in the urine. Drug clearance increases with postnatal age and decreases in the preterm and asphyxiated infant. Systemic absorption of oral doses is negligible; however, drug accumulation may occur with severe kidney impairment. Moderately plasma protein bound.

Monitoring serum drug concentrations is mandatory and should be done initially with the third dose. Adjust dosing regimen (dose or frequency) according to serum concentrations. Vancomycin serum concentrations decrease in a biphasic manner. The initial δ-phase represents drug distribution into the tissues; the serum concentration decreases rapidly. The β-phase represents total body elimination; the serum level decreases slowly. This is important because serum concentrations must be drawn during the β-phase (1 hour after completion of a 1-hour drug infusion). Target peak serum concentration: 25–30 mcg/ml (this is a post dose value; true peak serum concentration is actually higher).

Target trough concentration: 5–10 mcg/ml.

Cautions

Ototoxicity (with hearing loss) due to high serum levels and nephrotoxicity with proteinuria and transient increases in BUN and serum creatinine can occur.

Rapid IV infusion can cause histamine release with erythematous, pruritic rash over the upper body and face and rarely, tachycardia and hypotension (called Red Neck syndrome).

Hypersensitivity reactions with rash, fever, and leukopenia can occur. Can cause local irritation and necrosis at injection site.

Use may result in overgrowth of nonsusceptible organisms.

Use with caution in infants with kidney dysfunction; drug will accumulate.

Solution Compatibility

D5W, D10W, 0.9% NaCl, TPN without heparin.

Additive Compatibility

Calcium gluconate, hydrocortisone, potassium chloride.

Additive Incompatibility

Aminophylline, chloramphenicol, heparin, phenobarbital, sodium bicarbonate.

Drug Interactions

Aminoglycosides (amikacin, gentamicin, tobramycin): concurrent use may potentiate nephrotoxicity of aminoglycosides.

Ototoxic drugs (amikacin, furosemide, gentamicin, tobramycin): additive ototoxicity possible with concurrent use of other ototoxic drugs.

Nursing Considerations

- Obtain culture and sensitivity studies prior to initiation of therapy.
- CAREFUL attention to dose scheduling when q 18 hour interval is used.
- Infuse slowly IV over 1 hour.
- Monitor HR and BP during infusion
- Observe IV site for extravasation.
- Monitor kidney function.
- Consider audiometric testing (brainstem auditory evoked responses) prior to infant's discharge.

- Monitor serum drug concentrations, initially with the third dose and as indicated by changes in infant's condition or with changes in drug dosing:
  - trough: obtain blood 15 minutes before the third dose.
  - peak: obtain blood 1 hour after completion of a 1-hour IV infusion of drug (this is actually a post-dose value).

Antifungals

Amphotericin B

Brand Name

Fungizone

Forms

Injection 50 mg vial (for reconstitution).

Uses

Antifungal. Treatment of systemic infections caused by susceptible strains of *Candida* and other fungi. Frequently used in combination with flucytosine.

Dose

Initial dose: 0.1 mg/kg IV infusion. One dose.
Day 2 0.2 mg/kg IV infusion. One dose.
Day 3 0.4 mg/kg IV infusion. One dose.
Maintenance: 0.5 mg/kg IV infusion q 24 hours for 4–6 weeks.
Administer q 48 hours in infants that are anuric.

Pharmacokinetics

Fungicidal and fungistatic. Poorly absorbed from the GI tract. Poor CSF penetration (3% of serum concentration). Intrathecal route necessary to treat CNS infections. Half-life is approximately 2 weeks with long-term administration. Details of metabolism and elimination are unknown (only 3% eliminated unchanged in the urine). Highly plasma protein bound (>90%).

Cautions

Nephrotoxicity with decreased renal blood flow, decreased glomerular filtration rate, and renal tubular acidosis is common. Renal tubular acidosis can cause potassium and magnesium loss via the kidneys with resulting hypokalemia and hypomagnesemia. Hematotoxicity with bone marrow suppression, anemia (normocytic and normochromic), thrombocytopenia, and rarely, agranulocytosis can occur. Vomiting, fever, chills, and rarely, hypotension (during infusion), cardiac arrhythmias, and liver damage can occur. Thrombophlebitis and irritation at injection site are common.

Use with caution in infants with kidney dysfunction.

Solution Compatibility

D5W, D10W.

Solution Incompatibility

Do NOT mix with electrolyte (will precipitate drug) or bacteriostatic solutions. Reconstitute with nonpreserved sterile water.

Additive Compatibility

Do NOT mix with other drugs except heparin.

Drug Interactions

Aminoglycosides (amikacin, gentamicin, tobramycin): increased risk of nephrotoxicity.

Digoxin: frequency of cardiac arrhythmias due to digoxin may be increased.

Diuretics that waste potassium: thiazide diuretics and furosemide may cause serious loss of serum potassium when used in a patient receiving amphotericin B.

Nursing Considerations

- Obtain culture and sensitivity studies prior to initiation of therapy.
- Administer once daily by slow IV infusion over 4–6 hours.
- Use controlled infusion device for administration.
- Final concentration of drug infusion should be 0.1 mg/ml.
- In-line filter should have a pore diameter greater than 1 μm.
- Observe IV site closely, before and during infusion, for signs of phlebitis.
- Monitor HR and rhythm and BP during infusion.
- Monitor infant's temperature. Consider prophylactic administration of acetaminophen.
- Monitor serum electrolytes (especially potassium).
- Monitor CBC and platelet count.
- Monitor kidney function and urine output.
- Monitor liver function.

Anti-Infectives

Flucytosine

Brand Name

Ancobon

Forms

Capsules 250 mg, 500 mg (can be made into oral suspension).

Uses

Antifungal. Treatment of infections caused by susceptible fungi including *Candida* and *Cryptococcus*.
Not used as a single agent because fungal resistance develops quickly.
Frequently used in combination with amphotericin B.

Dose

12.5–37.5 mg/kg/dose PO q 6 hours.
Adjust dosing interval in infants with kidney impairment.
Moderate kidney impairment (<50%) q 8–12 hours.
Severe kidney impairment (<10%) q 24 hours.

Pharmacokinetics

Well absorbed from the GI tract (75–90%). Distributes widely into body fluids and tissues. Excellent CSF penetration with drug concentration 60–100% of serum levels. Half-life is up to 6 hours with normal kidney function. Almost totally eliminated unchanged in the urine with only minimal amounts of the drug metabolized.
Therapeutic serum level (peak): 50–75 mcg/ml.

Cautions

Adverse reactions occur with serum levels >100 mcg/ml. Flucytosine is a pro-drug metabolized by susceptible fungi to the active compound fluorouracil (an antimetabolite used in chemotherapy). Side effects similar to chemotherapeutic agents are possible: bone marrow suppression (with anemia, leukopenia, thrombocytopenia, and rarely, agranulocytosis), vomiting, diarrhea, abdominal distention, and rash. Can also cause reversible liver injury (increased SGOT, SGPT, alkaline phosphatase).

Use with caution in infants with kidney dysfunction or hematologic disorder. Contraindicated in infants that are anuric.

Drug Interactions

Aminoglycosides (amikacin, gentamicin, tobramycin): may impair kidney function and reduce clearance of flucytosine, with possible increased plasma levels of flucytosine and toxicity.
Amphotericin B: see "*Aminoglycosides.*"
Vancomycin: see "*Aminoglycosides.*"

Nursing Considerations

- Refer to drug information provided by manufacturer (with drug).
- Obtain culture and sensitivity studies prior to initiation of therapy.
- Shake oral suspension well before drawing up dose.
- Monitor CBC and platelet count (establish baseline values).

Anti-Infectives

- Monitor kidney function and urine output (interferes with some methods of creatinine determinations—see manufacturer's drug information).
- Monitor flucytosine serum levels. Obtain peak level 2 hours after PO administration.
- Monitor liver function.
- Observe infant for GI disturbances: vomiting, gastric residuals, abdominal distention, and pain. Can mimic necrotizing enterocolitis.

Nystatin

Brand Names

Mycostatin, Nystex, Nilstat, various

Forms

Oral suspension 100,000 units/ml in 60 ml bottle (contains paraben preservatives).
Topical cream and ointment 100,000 units/gm in 15 gm and 30 gm tubes.

Uses

Antifungal. Treatment and prevention of infections of the skin, mucous membranes, and intestinal tract caused by *Candida*.
Oral suspension and topical ointment have been used in combination to treat candidal diaper rash.

Dose

Oral suspension: 1–2 ml/dose PO q 6–8 hours. Swab mouth q 6–8 hours in the small preterm infant.
Topical preparation: apply thin coat to affected area q 6 hours.

Continue treatment for 48–72 hours after candidiasis has cleared to prevent recurrence of infection.

Pharmacokinetics

Fungicidal and fungistatic. Oral preparation is poorly absorbed from the GI tract. Topical preparation is not absorbed with intact skin and mucous membranes. Oral suspension is almost entirely eliminated unchanged in the feces.

Cautions

Hypersensitivity with rash, fever, and eosinophilia is very rare. Vomiting and diarrhea can occur with administration of oral suspension. Constituents of the topical preparation (ethylenediamine, parabens, and thimerosal) can cause contact dermatitis.

Nursing Considerations

- Shake oral suspension well before drawing up dose.
- Administer oral suspension with syringe, dropper, or swab into the sides of mouth.
- Administer after feeding. Presence of food in mouth can deactivate drug.
- Change infant's pacifier daily to minimize recurrence of infection.
- Observe for diarrhea.
- Apply thin coat of topical cream or ointment to affected skin area.
- Keep affected skin area clean and dry.
- Osmolality (Nilstat): 2605 mOsm/kg H_2O (FP).

Antivirals

Acyclovir

Brand Name

Zovirax

Forms

Injection 500 mg vial (for reconstitution).

Uses

Antiviral. Treatment of systemic infections, especially encephalitis, caused by herpes simplex Types 1 and 2 (HSV-1 and HSV-2) and varicella-zoster.

Dose

5–15 mg/kg/dose IV q 8 hours for 10 days.
Increase dosing interval in infants with kidney impairment.

Pharmacokinetics

Distributes widely throughout body tissues and fluids. Penetrates well into CSF (up to 50% of serum concentration). Acyclovir is a "pro-drug" that is preferentially taken up and converted to its active form by the virus-infected cells. Half-life is about 4 hours and is related to degree of kidney function and maturity. Eliminated mainly as unchanged drug in the urine with only about 15% of the drug metabolized. Drug will accumulate with kidney impairment.

Cautions

Toxicity is rare because the drug is preferentially taken up by infected cells. Transient decrease in kidney function (with crystalluria, increased BUN, serum creatinine, and decreased creatinine clearance) can occur. Risk of adverse kidney effects depends on degree of infant's hydration, urine output, rate of drug administration, and concomitant use of other nephrotoxic drugs. Very rarely bone marrow suppression (with leukopenia and thrombocytopenia), liver impairment (with a transient increase in SGOT, SGPT, and alkaline phosphatase), and CNS effects (with lethargy, obtundation, tremors, or agitation) may occur. Irritation, pain, and phlebitis at injection site is common.

Use with caution in infants with kidney dysfunction or fluid restrictions.

Solution Compatibility

D5W, D10W, 0.9% NaCl.

Additive Compatibility

Do NOT mix with other drugs.
Do NOT mix with biologic (blood, platelets) and/or colloidal fluids (human serum albumin, plasma protein fraction).

Drug Interactions

Aminoglycosides (amikacin, gentamicin, tobramycin): concurrent use can potentiate nephrotoxicity of acyclovir.
Vancomycin: see "*Aminoglycosides.*"

Nursing Considerations

• Obtain culture and sensitivity studies prior to initiation of therapy.

- Infuse slowly IV over 1 hour.
- Use controlled infusion device for administration.
- Final concentration of infusion should be ≤7 mg/ml.
- Observe IV site closely for phlebitis (further dilution of drug may decrease irritation).
- Provide adequate hydration and maintain adequate urine output (>2 ml/kg/hr).
- Monitor kidney function and urine output.
- Monitor CBC and platelet count.
- Monitor liver function.
- Monitor infant's CNS status (note lethargy, obtundation, tremors, or agitation).
- Refrigeration of acyclovir in solution may cause precipitation, which will redissolve at room temperature without loss of potency.

Ribavirin

Brand Name

Virazole

Forms

Inhalation 6 gm vial (for reconstitution).

Uses

Antiviral. Treatment of pulmonary infections caused by respiratory syncytial virus (RSV) or influenza A virus (various strains).

Dose

Administered as an aerosol over 8–12 hours daily for 3–7 days. Do not exceed 7 days of therapy.

The 6 gm vial of drug is initially reconstituted with 50–100 ml sterile water for injection or inhalation (additive free) and then is further diluted to a final volume of 300 ml (20 mg/ml). The drug is delivered from the Small Particle Aerosol Generator (Model SPAG-2). The Model SPAG-2 by Viratek will accept 300 ml of the final concentration (20 mg/ml), and the aerosol will last for 12–24 hours. The actual dose received depends upon the infant's respiratory rate, tidal volume, and the duration of the aerosol.

The aerosol is ideally administered via an oxygen hood; however, the use of an oxygen tent or facet mask is acceptable. Do NOT administer to infants requiring assisted ventilation. The drug may crystallize in, and obstruct, the ET tube and ventilator equipment and compromise ventilation and gas exchange (see "NOTE" under "Nursing Considerations").

Pharmacokinetics

Currently, the kinetics of ribavirin have only been studied in a small number of patients. Ribavirin is absorbed systemically with aerosol administration. Highest drug concentration is in the respiratory tract and red blood cells. The drug penetrates CSF after chronic oral use (experimentally), but penetration is delayed and would probably not be significant with a 3–5 day course of aerosol therapy. Half-life in pediatric patients is about 10 hours, with the half-life in the airways about 1.5–2.5 hours. Metabolism to the active antiviral compound 1,2,4-triazole-3-carboxamide probably occurs in the liver. Metabolite and unchanged drug are eliminated primarily in the urine. Little, if any, drug appears to be eliminated in expired CO_2.

Cautions

Can cause mild, reversible anemia and transient increase in serum bilirubin, SGOT and SGPT with IV or PO use and reticulocytosis, rash, and conjunctivitis (which may also affect health care personnel if mist escapes oxygen hood) with aerosol use. In severely ill infants with underlying life-threatening conditions, inhalation of drug has been associated with bronchospasm aggravation and worsening of respiratory function, apnea. Bacterial pneumonia, pneumothorax, ventilator dependency, digoxin toxicity, hypotension, and cardiac arrest have been observed in patients receiving ribavirin. Mutagenic in mammalian cell experiments. Teratogenic and/or embryocidal in animal species. Pregnant women and women of childbearing age should avoid exposure to ribavirin aerosol.

Use with caution in infants receiving digoxin.

Use with caution in infants requiring assisted ventilation.

Nursing Considerations

- Obtain viral culture prior to initiation of therapy.
- Review operator's manual for Model SPAG-2 provided by the manufacturer.
- Do NOT administer using any other aerosol generator.
- Do NOT administer concomitantly with other drug solutions for nebulization.
- Check delivery apparatus for particulate matter and discoloration (leaves white, crystalline residue).

- Ribavirin should only be administered by experienced personnel trained in the use of the specialized equipment necessary to administer the drug.
- Monitor infant's respiratory status closely during administration (respiratory effort, pulse oximetry, TcO_2, $TcCO_2$, and blood gases).
- Monitor reticulocyte count.
- Do NOT allow pregnant or breast-feeding women to enter room where ribavirin aerosol is being administered.

NOTE NOT recommended by the manufacturer for use in infants requiring assisted ventilation. Mechanical problems caused by the precipitation of the drug in ventilator equipment, including the ETT, may result in ineffective and unsafe assisted ventilation with inadequate gas exchange and possible obstruction of gas flow leading to increased PEEP and/or PIP and an increased risk of barotrauma. However, if the benefits outweigh the risks, ribavirin can be used in infants requiring assisted ventilation; the AAP recommends the use of a breathing circuit filter to avoid mechanical problems with ventilatory equipment. A breathing circuit filter is inserted in the expiratory line of the ventilator circuit in front of the expiratory valve and in the inspiratory line between the humidifier and the one-way, T-shaped value through which the solution for nebulization enters. The breathing circuit filters should be changed routinely, and the ETT and connecting sites should be checked periodically for precipitated drug.

Chapter 8

Corticosteroids

Corticosteroids are hormones, produced and secreted by the adrenal cortex, or their semisynthetic derivatives. Steroids have multiple effects on various organs and consequently produce many unneeded and often unwanted side effects. Corticosteroids are described as glucocorticoids or mineralocorticoids depending upon the hormone's ability to affect fluid and electrolyte balance in the distal renal tubules. Corticosteroids used as anti-inflammatory agents are glucocorticoids.

Relative Anti-inflammatory Activity:

Drug	Approximate Equivalent Dose	Duration of Activity	Anti-inflammatory Activity
	mg	*hrs*	
Hydrocortisone	20	6–12	+
Prednisone	5	12–36	+ +
Methylprednisolone	4	12–36	+ +
Dexamethasone	0.75	36–54	+ + + +

Corticosteroids have limited applications in neonatal medicine. Uses include: anti-inflammatory, reduction of airway edema, adjunct to weaning mechanical ventilation and possible prevention of severe

bronchopulmonary dysplasia, treatment of refractory
neonatal hypoglycemia, treatment of Gram-negative
septic shock, and replacement therapy in adrenal
insufficiency.

Dexamethasone

Brand Names

Decadron, Hexadrol, various

Forms

Injection 4 mg/ml in 1 ml and 5 ml vials (may contain
benzyl alcohol or parabens).
Elixir 0.1 mg/ml (contains alcohol 5%) in 120 ml bottle.

Uses

Anti-inflammatory. Used to reduce airway edema
before and after tracheal extubation and to facilitate
weaning of mechanical ventilation in infants with early
stages of bronchopulmonary dysplasia. Long-acting
corticosteroid.

Dose

Reduction of airway edema 0.5 mg/kg/dose IV q 6
hours × 3 doses.
Administer first dose 6 hours prior to extubation.
To facilitate weaning of mechanical ventilation (Avery
GB, et al.):

  0.25 mg/kg/dose IV, PO q 12 hours × 3 days, then
  0.15 mg/kg/dose IV, PO q 12 hours × 3 days, then
  decrease dose by 10% every 3 days until a dose of
  0.05 mg/kg/dose IV, PO q 12 hours × 3 days is given.

Then give 0.05 mg/kg/dose IV, PO qod × 3 doses, then discontinue.

Pharmacokinetics

Well absorbed from the GI tract after PO administration. Rapid onset of action. Duration of activity is 36–54 hours. Glucocorticoids are reduced, primarily in the liver, to their active form. Metabolized in the liver and most tissues and then excreted in the urine, and small amounts in the bile, with some unmetabolized drug.

Cautions

Prolonged use may cause adrenal insufficiency by suppression of the hypothalamic-pituitary-adrenal axis (HPA axis). Most significant complication of therapy is the increased risk of sepsis due to the suppression of the immune system. Drug may also mask signs of sepsis. Sodium and water retention (less with dexamethasone than most steroids), hypertension, hypokalemia, hypocalcemia, glucose intolerance with hyperglycemia and glycosuria, and hypercholesterolemia can occur. Vomiting, diarrhea or constipation, abdominal distention, and GI ulceration and/or bleeding may also occur. The efficacy of prophylactic use of H-2 antagonists (cimetidine and ranitidine) or antacids in preventing GI bleeding has not been proven.

Prolonged use may also cause osteoporosis, retarded bone growth, muscle wasting, and delayed wound healing.

Acute or too rapid withdrawal of drug after prolonged use (>7 days) can cause acute adrenal insufficiency with fever, hypotension, hypoglycemia, and shock.

Use with caution in infants with kidney dysfunction, hypothyroidism, or heart disease. CONTRAINDICATED in infants with untreated systemic infections.

Solution Compatibility

D5W, D10W, 0.9% NaCl.

Additive Compatibility

Amikacin, aminophylline, cimetidine, nafcillin.

Additive Incompatibility

Vancomycin.

Drug Interactions

Amphotericin B: increased risk of potassium loss and hypokalemia with concurrent use.
Furosemide: see "*Amphotericin B*."
Hydrochlorothiazide: see "*Amphotericin B*."
Phenobarbital: effects of corticosteroids may be decreased. Effects of interaction may occur for several days after phenobarbital is discontinued.
Phenytoin: see "*Phenobarbital*." Effects of phenytoin may be altered; may increase or decrease plasma levels.
Rifampin: see "*Phenobarbital*." Effects of interaction may occur for several days after rifampin is discontinued.
Vaccines/toxoids: dexamethasone may decrease immune response to vaccines and toxoids.

Nursing Considerations

- Infuse slowly IV over 10–15 minutes.
- Monitor BP.
- Monitor serum electrolytes, calcium, and cholesterol.
- Monitor blood and urine glucose.
- Monitor kidney function and urine output.
- Check infant's stool and gastric contents for occult and gross blood.
- Monitor daily weights.
- Observe for signs of sepsis: increased ventilatory and/or oxygen requirements, increased apnea, temperature instability, feeding intolerance, decreased activity, and abnormalities on regularly monitored CBC.
- Osmolality (Hexadrol 0.1 mg/ml): 5415 mOsm/kg H_2O (FP).

NOTE Ineffective as replacement therapy for adrenal insufficiency because its mineralocorticoid activity is low.

Hydrocortisone

Brand Names

Solu-Cortef, various

Forms

Injection 100 mg vials, and others (for reconstitution; may contain benzyl alcohol).

Uses

Anti-inflammatory. Used to increase gluconeogenesis and decrease glucose utilization in refractory neonatal hypoglycemia; used in the management of Gram-negative septic shock (controversial); used for replacement therapy of adrenal insufficiency. Short-acting corticosteroid.

Dose

Neonatal hypoglycemia 1–4 mg/kg/dose IV q 8 hours.
Adrenal insufficiency 1 mg/kg/dose IV, PO q 24 hours.

Pharmacokinetics

Rapid onset of action. Duration of activity is 6–12 hours. Glucocorticoids are reduced, primarily in the liver, to their active form. Metabolized in the liver and most tissues and then excreted in the urine, and small amounts in the bile, with some unmetabolized drug.

Cautions

Prolonged use may cause adrenal insufficiency by suppression of the hypothalamic-pituitary-adrenal axis (HPA axis). Most significant complication of therapy is the increased risk of sepsis due to the suppression of the immune system. Drug may also mask signs of sepsis. Sodium and water retention (hydrocortisone > dexamethasone), hypertension, hypokalemia, hypocalcemia, glucose intolerance with hyperglycemia and glycosuria, and hypercholesterolemia can occur. Vomiting, diarrhea or constipation, abdominal distention, and GI ulceration and/or bleeding may also occur. The efficacy of prophylactic use of H-2 antagonists (cimetidine and ranitidine) or antacids in preventing GI bleeding has not been proven.

Prolonged use may also cause osteoporosis,

retarded bone growth, muscle wasting, and delayed wound healing.

Acute or too rapid withdrawal of drug after prolonged use (>7 days) can cause acute adrenal insufficiency with fever, hypotension, hypoglycemia, and shock.

Use with caution in infants with kidney dysfunction, hypothyroidism, or heart disease. CONTRAINDICATED in infants with untreated systemic infections.

Solution Compatibility

D5W, D10W, D20W, 0.9% NaCl.

Additive Compatibility

Amikacin, aminophylline, amphotericin B, calcium chloride, calcium gluconate, chloramphenicol, clindamycin, penicillin G, piperacillin, potassium chloride, vancomycin.

Additive Incompatibility

Ampicillin, hydralazine, lidocaine, methicillin, metronidazole, phenobarbital.

Drug Interactions

Amphotericin B: increased risk of potassium loss and hypokalemia with concurrent use.
Furosemide: see "*Amphotericin B.*"
Hydrochlorothiazide: see "Amphotericin B."
Phenobarbital: effects of corticosteroids may be decreased. Effects of interaction may occur for several days after phenobarbital is discontinued.
Phenytoin: see "*Phenobarbital.*" Effects of phenytoin

may be altered; may increase or decrease plasma levels.

Rifampin: see *"Phenobarbital."* Effects of interaction may occur for several days after rifampin is discontinued.

Vaccines/toxoids: hydrocortisone may decrease immune response to vaccines and toxoids.

Nursing Considerations

- Infuse slowly IV over 10–15 minutes.
- Monitor BP.
- Monitor serum electrolytes, calcium, and cholesterol.
- Monitor blood and urine glucose.
- Monitor kidney function and urine output.
- Check infant's stool and gastric contents for occult and gross blood.
- Monitor daily weights.
- Observe for signs of sepsis: increased ventilatory and/or oxygen requirements, increased apnea, temperature instability, feeding intolerance, decreased activity, and abnormalities on regularly monitored CBC.

Chapter 9

Vitamins, Minerals, and Electrolytes

Vitamins

Folic Acid

Brand Names

Folvite, various

Forms

Injection 5 mg/ml (contains benzyl alcohol). Diluted with nonpreserved sterile water to formulate PO preparation 50 mcg/ml.

Uses

Essential for erythropoiesis.
Dietary supplement for the preterm infant who has low folic acid stores at birth and a high utilization rate due to rapid growth. Water-soluble vitamin.

Dose

50 mcg (to 100 mcg)/day PO.
Usual liquid multivitamin preparations do not contain folic acid.
Start when enteral feedings are established and continue until there is adequate intake with human milk or

formula (300 ml/day) or until infant reaches a weight of ~2 kg (see Table 9.1).

Deficiency

Mild forms of deficiency are manifested by low serum folate levels and hypersegmentation of neutrophils. Severe deficiency may result in megaloblastic anemia, usually occuring at 6–10 weeks of age in the preterm infant.

Pharmacokinetics

Rapidly absorbed from the GI tract (mainly in the proximal portion of the small intestine) after PO administration. Largely metabolized in the liver and excreted in the feces with very small amounts in the urine. About half of the total body folate stores are in the liver.

Cautions

Relatively nontoxic with recommended doses.

Drug Interactions

Phenytoin: reduced plasma levels and therapeutic effectiveness of phenytoin can occur.
Trimethoprim: may alter the metabolism of folic acid.

Nursing Considerations

• Monitor CBC and reticulocyte count.

Vitamin D$_2$ (Ergocalciferol)

Brand Names

Drisdol, Calciferol (contains propylene glycol)

Table 9.1.
Nutrient Content of Premature Infant Formulas and Human Milk (Units per 100 kcal)

	Human Milk	Mead Johnson Enfamil Premature	Ross Similac Special Care	Wyeth SMA Preemie	Ross Similac LBW
Vitamin A, IU	310	1200	680	300	300
Vitamin D, IU	3.05	330	150	60	60
Vitamin E, IU	0.32	4.6	4	1.9	3
Vitamin K, mcg	0.29	13	12	8.6	8
Vitamin C, mg	5.56	35	37	8.6	12
Folic acid, mcg	6.94	35	37	12.5	15
Calcium, mg	38.89	117	180	90	90
Phosphorus, mg	19.44	59	90	50	70
Calcium/phosphorous	2:1	2:1	2:1	1.8:1	1.3:1
Iron, mg	0.04	0.25	0.37	0.38	0.37
kcal/oz	21.3	20, 24	20, 24	24	24

Memory Bank for Neonatal Drugs

Forms

Drops 400 IU/0.05 ml (8000 IU/ml) in 60 ml bottles.

Uses

Essential for optimal calcium and phosphorus absorption and metabolism and for normal bone growth and calcification.
Dietary supplement for the prevention and treatment of bone disease (osteopenia and rickets) in the preterm infant. Fat-soluble vitamin.

Dose

400 IU (up to 1000 IU)/day PO.
Multivitamin preparations for infants contain 400 IU/ml.
See Table 9.1.

Deficiency

Deficiency can cause osteopenia and rickets.

Pharmacokinetics

Readily absorbed from the GI tract (intestines) if fat absorption is normal. Presence of bile is important for absorption. Metabolized in the liver and kidneys, with metabolites excreted primarily in the bile and feces.

Cautions

Toxicity can cause hypercalcemia with poor appetite, vomiting, diarrhea or constipation, abdominal cramps, drowsiness, hypotonia, and later, impaired kidney function (with polyuria and proteinuria), weight loss, growth retardation, and rarely, hypertension and car-

diac arrhythmias. Drug preparation is very
hyperosmolar and can cause GI irritation.

Use with caution in infants with hypoparathyroidism
or in infants receiving digoxin.

Drug Interactions

Digoxin: potential hypercalcemia with resulting
cardiac arrhythmias can occur.

Nursing Considerations

- AAP Committee on Nutrition RDA: 400 IU (for
  preterm and term infants).
- Administer with feeding to decrease GI irritation.
- Observe for signs of GI irritation: vomiting, gastric
  residuals, abdominal distention, diarrhea, gastric
  residuals or stools positive for occult blood.
- Provide adequate calcium and phosphorus intake.
- Monitor serum calcium and phosphorus.
- Attention to potential for fractures in infants with
  rickets.
- Protect drug from light and air.
- Osmolality (Drisdol): 20,460 mOsm/kg H_2O (FP).

Vitamin E (d,l-∂-Tocopherol)

Brand Name

Aquasol E

Forms

Drops 50 IU/ml (contains propylene glycol) in 12 ml
and 30 ml bottles.

Uses

Antioxidant. Preserves integrity of red cell wall and protects against hemolysis. Dietary supplement for the prevention and treatment of hemolytic anemia in the preterm infant who has low vitamin E stores at birth (till 3 months of age), decreased absorption, and higher requirements due to rapid growth. Water-soluble vitamin.

Dose

5–30 IU/day PO.
Multivitamin preparations for infants contain 5 IU/ml. Start when enteral feedings are established and continue for the first 2–3 months of life (see Table 9.1).

Deficiency

Deficiency can cause mild hemolytic anemia, reticulocytosis, mild generalized edema, and irritability, usually occurring at 6–8 weeks of age. Elevated platelet count ($>250,000/mm^3$) with eosinophilia may indicate vitamin E deficiency. Deficiency can be exacerbated by early administration of iron supplements or high iron intake.

Pharmacokinetics

Absorption from the GI tract depends on the presence of bile. Metabolized in the liver and excreted primarily in the bile and feces with small amounts in the urine. Stored in adipose tissue.

Cautions

Usually nontoxic with recommended doses. Necrotizing enterocolitis has occurred with administration of high doses. Drug preparation is hyperosmolar and can cause GI irritation with abdominal cramping and diarrhea.

Drug Interactions

Iron preparations: concomitant administration of iron preparation decreases intestinal absorption of vitamin E supplement. Vitamin E may decrease response to iron therapy.

Nursing Considerations

- AAP Committee on Nutrition RDA: 5–25 IU of supplemental oral vitamin E (for preterm infants).
- Administer with feeding to decrease GI irritation.
- Observe for signs of GI irritation: vomiting, diarrhea, abdominal distention, gastric residuals or stools positive for occult blood.
- Monitor hematocrit and reticulocyte count.
- Observe for signs of anemia in the preterm infant: pale color, decreased activity, recurrent apnea, poor weight gain, tachycardia, tachypnea or dyspnea.
- Protect drug from air and light.
- Osmolality (Aquasol E): 3990 mOsm/kg H_2O (FP).

Vitamin K₁ (Phytonadione)

Brand Name

AquaMEPHYTON

Forms

Injection 2 mg/ml (contains benzyl alcohol).

Uses

Prevention and treatment of hemorrhagic disease of the newborn.

Dose

0.5–1 mg IM (one dose) at birth.
Treatment of severe hemorrhagic disease: 1–2 mg (up to 10 mg) IV prn.
Prophylaxis for infants receiving TPN: 1 mg/week IM, IV.

Deficiency

Classic hemorrhagic disease of the newborn occurs between 2 and 10 days of age and is manifested by generalized ecchymoses or GI hemorrhage, and bleeding from the umbilical stump or circumcision; it occurs most commonly in breast-fed infants who did not receive vitamin K prophylaxis at birth. The "late onset" (>2 weeks of age) form of hemorrhagic disease of the newborn is more common and is manifested by intracranial hemorrhage; again, it occurs most commonly in breast-fed infants who did not receive vitamin K at birth.

Pharmacokinetics

Mechanisms of metabolism and excretion are unknown.

Cautions

Rapid IV administration can cause seizure-like activity, tachycardia, brief hypotension, cardiac irregularities, flushing, bronchospasm, shock, and respiratory and/or cardiac arrest and death. Can cause pain and swelling at IM injection site.

Solution Compatibilities

Dextrose-saline combinations, D5W, D10W, 0.45% NaCl, 0.9% NaCl, TPN.

Nursing Considerations

- Use anterolateral thigh for IM administration.
- AVOID administration by IV push. Administer slowly IV at <1 mg/minute.
- AAP recommends prophylatic administration of vitamin K to all newborns at birth.
- Monitor prothrombin time in infants with hemorrhagic disease.
- Protect drug from light.

Vitamins, Multiple

Brand Names

Poly-Vi-Sol, Vi-Daylin, various

Forms

Drops 1 ml contains vitamin A 1500 IU, vitamin C 35 mg, vitamin D 400 IU, vitamin E 5 IU, and also thiamine, riboflavin, niacin, vitamin B_6, and vitamin B_{12} (contains preservatives).

Uses

Dietary supplement for the preterm and term infant.
Fat-soluble and water-soluble vitamins.

Dose

1 ml/day PO.
Start when enteral feedings are established (see
Table 9.1).

Cautions

Drug preparation is very hyperosmolar and can cause
GI irritation with vomiting and/or gastric residuals.

Nursing Considerations

- Provides 100% of the U.S. RDA for infants (only
  75% U.S. RDA of vitamin B_{12}).
- Administer with feeding to decrease GI irritation.
- Observe for signs of GI irritation: vomiting, gastric
  residuals, abdominal distention, diarrhea, gastric
  residuals or stools positive for occult blood.
- Divide daily dose if infant exhibits intolerance
  (vomiting, gastric residuals).
- Osmolality (Poly-Vi-Sol): 11,180 mOsm/kg H_2O (FP).

Minerals

Calcium Chloride 10%

Brand Names

Various

Forms

Injection 100 mg/ml (27 mg [1.36 mEq] Ca^{2+}/ml) in 10
ml ampuls, vials, and prefilled syringes.

Uses

Treatment of hypocalcemia (total serum calcium <7 mg/dl or ionized calcium <2.4 mg/dl).
Used to antagonize cardiotoxic effects of hyperkalemia.

Dose

0.35–0.7 ml (9.5–19 mg Ca^{2+})/kg/dose IV.

Pharmacokinetics

Onset of action is within minutes. Drug is in ionized form and is readily available, requiring no metabolism. Excreted in feces and urine.

Cautions

Rapid IV infusion can cause severe bradycardia, hypotension, arrhythmias, sustained myocardial contraction, and asystole. More hyperosmolar than calcium gluconate. Extravasation of IV injection can cause local tissue necrosis and sloughing. Administration of large doses or use in infants with kidney impairment can result in hypercalcemia (>12 mg/dl) with vomiting, poor feeding, hypotonia, lethargy, polyuria, hypertension, and seizures.

Use with caution in digitalized infants and in infants with heart disease or kidney dysfunction.

Solution Compatibility

Compatible with most IV solutions, including fat emulsion 10%.

Additive Compatibility

Amikacin, chloramphenicol, lidocaine, methicillin, penicillin G.

Additive Incompatibility

Amphotericin B, sodium bicarbonate, tobramycin.

Nursing Considerations

- AVOID overtreatment. Hypercalcemia may be more dangerous than hypocalcemia.
- Dilute at least 1 : 1 with compatible diluent.
- Infuse slowly IV over 30–60 minutes (over 5–10 minutes in the presence of severe cardiotoxic effects of hyperkalemia).
- Monitor HR, rhythm, and BP during IV infusion.
- Use large vein for administration.
- Observe IV site closely for extravasation. Treatment for extravasation: Hyaluronidase (Wydase) 150 unit vial reconstituted with 1 ml of NS. Infiltrate throughout affected area as soon as possible. Use 25 gauge needle.
- Do NOT administer IM.
- Monitor total serum and/or ionized calcium.
- Observe for signs of HYPOcalcemia: irritability, jitteriness, tremors, seizures, and apnea. Changes in EKG include: prolonged QT_c interval.
- Observe for signs of HYPERcalcemia: vomiting, poor feeding, hypotonia, lethargy, polyuria, hypertension, and seizures. Changes in EKG include: shortened QT_c interval, prolonged PR interval and QRS duration, and arrhythmias (ventricular tachycardia, premature ventricular contractions, AV block).

Vitamins, Minerals, and Electrolytes　　　　**213**

Calcium Glubionate

Brand Name

Neo-Calglucon

Forms

Oral solution 360 mg/ml (23 mg [1.16 mEq] Ca^{2+}/ml) in pint bottles (contains preservatives).

Uses

Dietary supplement for the treatment and prevention of hypocalcemia in the enterally fed infant (total serum calcium <7 mg/dl or ionized calcium <2.4 mg/dl).

Dose

1.3–3.5 ml (30–80 mg Ca^{2+})/kg/day PO divided equally among feedings.
Dose is total intake, including PO feedings. Adjust dose as indicated by total serum or ionized calcium.

Pharmacokinetics

Well absorbed from the GI tract after PO administration. Rapidly incorporated into skeletal tissues with 99% of the body's calcium found in bone. Ionized calcium is the active fraction present in the plasma that exerts physiologic effects. Excreted mainly in the feces with small amounts in the urine.

Cautions

Hyperosmolar. Gastric irritation and osmotic diarrhea can occur. Administration of large doses or use in infants with kidney impairment can result in hypercalcemia (>12 mg/dl) with vomiting, poor feeding, hypotonia, lethargy, polyuria, hypertension, and seizures.

Use with caution in digitalized infants and in infants with heart disease or kidney dysfunction.

Nursing Considerations

- AVOID overtreatment. Hypercalcemia may be more dangerous than hypocalcemia.
- Administer with feeding (or after) to decrease gastric irritation.
- Observe for signs of gastric irritation: vomiting, gastric residuals, diarrhea, abdominal distention, gastric residuals or stools positive for occult blood.
- Monitor total serum and/or ionized calcium.
- Observe for signs of HYPOcalcemia: irritability, jitteriness, seizures, and apnea. Changes in EKG include: prolonged QT_c interval.
- Observe for signs of HYPERcalcemia: vomiting, poor feeding, hypotonia, lethargy, polyuria, hypertension, and seizures. Changes in EKG include: shortened QT_c interval, prolonged PR interval and QRS duration, and arrhythmias (ventricular tachycardia, premature ventricular contractions, AV block).
- Osmolality (Neo-Calglucon): 2455 mOsm/kg H_2O (FP).

Calcium Gluconate 10%

Brand Names

Various

Forms

Injection 100 mg/ml (9.4 mg [0.48 mEq] Ca^{2+}/ml) in 10 ml ampuls and vials.

Uses

Calcium salt of choice for the treatment and prevention of hypocalcemia (total serum calcium <7 mg/dl or ionized calcium <2.4 mg/dl).
Used to antagonize cardiotoxic effects of hyperkalemia.

Dose

1–2 ml (9–18 mg Ca^{2+})/kg/dose IV.
Maintenance 30–80 mg Ca^{2+}/kg/day IV intermittent or continuous infusion or PO divided equally among feedings. Dose is total intake, including PO feedings. Adjust dose as indicated by total serum or ionized calcium.

Pharmacokinetics

Well absorbed from the GI tract after PO administration. Rapidly incorporated into skeletal tissues with 99% of the body's calcium found in bone. Ionized calcium is the active fraction present in the plasma that exerts physiologic effects. Excreted mainly in the feces with small amounts in the urine.

Cautions

Rapid IV administration can cause severe bradycardia, hypotension, cardiac arrhythmias, and asystole. Extravasation of IV injection can cause local tissue necrosis and sloughing. Gastric irritation and constipation can occur with PO administration. Administration of large doses or use in infants with kidney impairment can result in hypercalcemia (>12 mg/dl) with vomiting, poor feeding, hypotonia, lethargy, polyuria, hypertension, and seizures.

Use with caution in digitalized infants and in infants with heart disease or kidney dysfunction.

Solution Compatibility

Compatible with most IV solutions, including TPN and fat emulsion 10%.

Additive Compatibility

Aminophylline, chloramphenicol, heparin, hydrocortisone, lidocaine, methicillin, penicillin G, phenobarbital, potassium chloride, vancomycin.

Additive Incompatibility

Amphotericin B, cefazolin, clindamycin, methylprednisolone, ± sodium bicarbonate, tobramycin. Also carbonates, phosphates, and sulfates.

Nursing Considerations

- AVOID overtreatment. Hypercalcemia may be more dangerous than hypocalcemia.
- May dilute 1:1 with compatible diluent.
- Infuse slowly IV over 30–60 minutes (over 5–10 minutes in the presence of severe cardiotoxic effects of hyperkalemia).
- Monitor HR, rhythm, and BP during bolus IV infusion.
- Observe IV site closely for extravasation. Treatment

Vitamins, Minerals, and Electrolytes   **217**

for extravasation: Hyaluronidase (Wydase) 150 unit vial reconstituted with 1 ml of NS. Infiltrate throughout affected area as soon as possible. Use 25 gauge needle.

- Do NOT administer IM.
- Administer PO with feeding.
- Observe for signs of gastric irritation and constipation: vomiting, gastric residuals, abdominal distention, visible loops of bowel, gastric residuals or stools positive for occult blood.
- Monitor total serum and/or ionized calcium.
- Observe for signs of HYPOcalcemia: irritability, jitteriness, tremors, seizures, and apnea. Changes in EKG include: prolonged QT_c interval.
- Observe for signs of HYPERcalcemia: vomiting, poor feeding, hypotonia, lethargy, polyuria, hypertension and seizures. Change in EKG include: shortened QT_c interval, prolonged PR interval and QRS duration, and arrhythmias (ventricular tachycardia, premature ventricular contractions, AV block).

Ferrous Sulfate

Brand Names

Fer-In-Sol, various

Forms

Drops 125 mg (25 mg elemental iron)/ml (contains alcohol).
Various oral solutions available.

Uses

Dietary supplement for the prevention and treatment of iron deficiency anemia in the preterm infant who has low iron stores at birth.

Dose

Prevention: 1–2 mg elemental iron/kg/day PO q 12–24 hours.
Treatment: 6 mg elemental iron/kg/day PO q 12–24 hours.
Administer as iron-fortified formula or therapeutic iron preparation. Start at ~2 months of age (when iron stores are usually depleted) and continue until 12–15 months of age (see Table 9.1).

Deficiency

Deficiency can cause anemia.

Pharmacokinetics

Absorption occurs along the entire length of the GI tract (mainly in the duodenum and proximal jejunum). Absorption depends on many factors including form and dose of iron, abundance of iron stores, and diet. Seventy per cent of iron is contained in hemoglobin, with 25% of iron stores mainly in the liver, reticuloendothelial system, spleen, and bone marrow. Most iron released by the destruction of hemoglobin is conserved and used by the body. Unabsorbed iron may be present in feces, causing black color.

Cautions

Acute overdose can cause acute GI irritation and pain, vomiting and diarrhea, green then tarry stools

Vitamins, Minerals, and Electrolytes   **219**

with blood, vomiting of blood, drowsiness, pallor, cyanosis, shock, and coma. Drug preparation is hyperosmolar and can cause gastric irritation and erosion, constipation, or diarrhea. Vitamin E deficiency hemolytic anemia can be exacerbated by early administration of iron or high iron doses.

Use with caution in infants <2 months of age.

Drug Interactions

Antacids: concurrent administration of antacids may decrease absorption of iron preparation.
Vitamin E: concurrent administration of iron preparation decreases intestinal absorption of vitamin E supplement. Vitamin E may decrease response to iron therapy.

Nursing Considerations

- AAP Committee on Nutrition RDA: 2 mg/kg/day (for preterm infants).
  1 mg/kg/day (for term infants).
  Start iron therapy no later than 2 months in the preterm infant and no later than 4 months in the term infant. Maximum daily dose not to exceed 15 mg.
- Provide adequate vitamin E intake for preterm infants prior to initiation of iron therapy.
- Administer with or after feedings to decrease GI irritation (maximum absorption occurs if administered between feedings).
- Observe for signs of GI irritation: vomiting, gastric residuals, abdominal distention, diarrhea or consti-

pation, gastric residuals or stools positive for occult blood.
- Monitor hematocrit and reticulocyte count.
- Observe for signs of anemia in the preterm infant: pale color, decreased activity, recurrent apnea, poor weight gain, tachycardia, tachypnea, or dyspnea.
- Consider use of iron-fortified formulas.
- Osmolality (Fer-In-Sol): 5010 mOsm/kg H_2O (FP).

Electrolytes

Arginine Hydrochloride

Brand Names

R-Gene

Forms

Injection 100 mg/ml (0.475 mEq Cl^-/ml) in 300 ml bottles.

Uses

Treatment and prevention of hypochloremia (serum chloride <95 mEq/L).

Dose

0.5–1 mEq Cl^-/kg/dose PO. Divide daily dose equally among feedings.
Dose and frequency dependent on serum chloride. Adjust dose as indicated.

Pharmacokinetics

Well absorbed from the GI tract after PO administration. Arginine is metabolized in the liver and is almost completely reabsorbed by the renal tubules. Chloride is excreted mainly by the kidneys.

Cautions

Low toxicity with PO administration. Large doses of chloride may cause a loss of bicarbonate with resultant metabolic acidosis. Increased serum creatinine and BUN may occur. Hyperosmolar. Can cause abdominal pain and distention.

Use with caution in infants with kidney dysfunction (potential for hyperkalemia) or acidosis.

Drug Interactions

Spironolactone: concurrent administration of potassium-sparing diuretics may increase risk of arginine-induced hyperkalemia.

Nursing Considerations

- Administer PO with feeding to decrease gastric irritation. Dilute with some formula or breast milk.
- Observe for signs of gastric irritation: vomiting, gastric residuals, diarrhea, abdominal distention, gastric residuals or stools positive for occult blood.
- Monitor serum chloride, potassium, and bicarbonate.
- Osmolality (injection 100 mg/ml): 950 mOsm/L.

Potassium Chloride

Brand Names

Various

Forms

Injection 2 mEq/ml in 10 ml and 20 ml ampuls, vials, and syringes. Various other injectables.
Oral solution 20% 40 mEq/15 ml (2.7 mEq/ml) in pint bottles (may contain alcohol). Various other oral solutions.

Uses

Potassium salt of choice for the treatment and prevention of hypokalemia (serum potassium <3–3.5 mEq/L).

Dose

Symptomatic hypokalemia 0.5–1 mEq/kg/dose SLOW IV infusion.
Maintenance 1–3 mEq/kg/day IV continuous infusion or PO in 2–4 divided doses.
Adjust dose as indicated by serum potassium concentration.

Pharmacokinetics

Slowly, but well absorbed from the GI tract after PO administration. Excreted mainly by the kidneys with small amounts excreted in the feces and by the skin. Losses are increased with vomiting and diarrhea.

Cautions

Hyperkalemia is the most common and most serious side effect. Large doses or rapid IV administration can cause hyperkalemia (>7 mEq/L) with hypotonia, cold skin, gray pallor, hypotension, cardiac arrhythmias, heart block, and possible asystole. Hyperosmolar. Extravasation of IV preparation can cause local tissue necrosis. Gastrointestinal irritation with vomiting, abdominal pain, and diarrhea can occur with PO administration. Alkalosis can decrease plasma levels, while acidosis can increase plasma levels.

Use with caution in digitalized infants and in infants with heart disease or kidney dysfunction. CONTRAIN-DICATED in infants with severe kidney dysfunction with oliguria or anuria.

Solution Compatibility

Dextrose-saline combinations, D5W, D10W, D20W, 0.45% NaCl, 0.9% NaCl, TPN.

Additive Compatibility

Compatible with most drugs.

Additive Incompatibility

Amphotericin B.

Drug Interactions

Spironolactone: concurrent administration of potassium-sparing diuretics may result in hyperkalemia with possible cardiac arrhythmias and asystole.
Captopril: hyperkalemia with possible cardiac arrhythmias and asystole may occur.

Nursing Considerations

- AVOID overtreatment. Hyperkalemia may be more dangerous than hypokalemia.
- Administer slowly IV over 1–2 hours. Do NOT administer by IV bolus.

- Monitor HR, rhythm, and BP during IV infusion.
- Do NOT administer IM.
- Administer PO preparation with feeding to decrease GI irritation. Dilute 20% oral solution in at least 10 ml of formula or breast milk.
- Observe for signs of GI irritation: vomiting, gastric residuals, diarrhea, abdominal distention, gastric residuals or stools positive for occult blood.
- Monitor serum potassium.
- Monitor kidney function and urine output.
- Observe for signs of HYPOkalemia: drowsiness, hypotonia, poor feeding, and tachycardia. Changes in EKG include: prolonged QT_c interval, depressed ST segment, flat or inverted T wave, appearance of U wave, prolonged PR interval, prominent P wave, and ectopic beats (supraventricular and ventricular). Digoxin (toxic) effects are enhanced in hypokalemia.
- Observe for signs of HYPERkalemia: hypotonia, cold skin, gray pallor, hypotension, cardiac arrhythmias, heart block, and possible asystole. Changes in EKG include: tall, peaked T waves (earliest manifestation), widening of QRS complex, PR and QT_c intervals, wide and flattened P waves, ectopic rhythms, and heart block. Effects are enhanced by hyponatremia, hypocalcemia, or acidosis.
- STOP all potassium administration in the presence of hyperkalemia.
- TREATMENT OF HYPERKALEMIA (>6.5 mEQ/L) WITHOUT CARDIAC SYMPTOMS: Sodium polystyrene sulfonate (Kayexalate) 1 gram/kg/dose PR, PO q 6 hours prn. Onset of action is within 1–2 hours. Each gram of drug removes 1

mEq potassium (exchanged for sodium). Monitor serum sodium and potassium and EKG.

- TREATMENT OF HYPERKALEMIA (>6.5 mEQ/L) WITH EARLY CARDIAC SYMPTOMS (PEAKED T WAVES):

  Sodium bicarbonate 1–2 mEq/kg/dose IV bolus over 5–10 minutes prn. Onset of action is within minutes. Facilitates shift of potassium into cells. Monitor serum sodium and potassium and EKG.

  OR

  Regular insulin 0.1–0.2 units /kg in glucose 400 mg/kg IV infusion over 30–60 minutes. Facilitates rapid shift of potassium into cells. Monitor blood glucose, serum potassium, and EKG. Utilize insulin:glucose ratio 1–2 units insulin:4 gm glucose.

  PLUS

  Sodium polystyrene sulfonate (Kayexalate) 1 gram/kg/dose PR, PO q 6 hours prn to remove excess potassium permanently.

- TREATMENT OF HYPERKALEMIA (>7–7.5 mEQ/L) WITH SEVERE CARDIAC SYMPTOMS:

  Calcium gluconate 10% 1–2 ml/kg/dose IV bolus infusion over 10 minutes prn. Onset of action is within minutes. Antagonizes the cardiac effects of potassium. Monitor serum calcium and potassium and EKG. Monitor HR, rhythm, and BP continuously during IV bolus infusion.

  PLUS

  Sodium polystyrene sulfonate (Kayexalate) 1 gram/kg/dose PR, PO q 6 hours prn to remove excess potassium permanently.

- Osmolality (injection 2 mEq/ml): 4355 mOsm/kg H_2O (FP).

Osmolality (oral solution 20 mEq/15 ml): 4370 mOsm/kg H_2O (FP).

Sodium Bicarbonate

Brand Names

Various

Forms

Injection 4.2% (0.5 mEq/ml) and 8.4% (1 mEq/ml) in syringes and vials.

Uses

Alkalinizing agent. Correction of documented metabolic acidosis (pH < 7.2) despite adequate ventilation.
Correction of bicarbonate deficit due to kidney and GI losses.

Dose

Metabolic Acidosis 1–2 mEq/kg/dose (2–4 ml/kg of 4.2% dilution) IV.
Doses should be based on pH, pCO_2, and base deficit:

$$\text{dose (mEq Na } HCO_3) = \text{weight (kg)} \times 0.3 \\ \times \text{ base deficit (mEq/ml)}$$

Kidney and GI Losses 2–3 mEq (to 10 mEq)/kg/day PO in 2–4 divided doses. Adjust dose as indicated by serum bicarbonate.

Pharmacokinetics

Rapid onset of action after IV administration. Duration of effect is 1–2 hours. Rapidly and well absorbed from

Vitamins, Minerals, and Electrolytes 227

the GI tract after PO administration. Rapidly metabolized in the liver and excreted in the urine.

Cautions

Excessive dosing, rapid rates of infusion, or use of concentrated solution can cause excessive increases in vascular volume, hypernatremia, hyperosmolality, hypercarbia (if inadequate ventilation), hypocalcemia, hypokalemia, and possibly intracranial hemorrhage. Severe alkalosis can cause hyperirritability, respiratory depression, and seizures. Can cause local tissue necrosis and/or sloughing with extravasation after IV administration. Gastric distention and flatulence can occur with PO administration.

Use with caution in infants with heart failure or severe kidney dysfunction and in infants receiving steroids.

Solution Compatibility

Dextrose-saline combinations, D5W, D10W, 0.45% NaCl, 0.9% NaCl.

Additive Compatibility

Amikacin, aminophylline, amphotericin B, chloramphenicol, cimetidine, clindamycin, heparin, lidocaine, nafcillin, oxacillin, potassium chloride.

Additive Incompatibility

Calcium chloride, calcium gluconate, epinephrine, magnesium sulfate, meperidine, methicillin, metoclopramide, morphine, penicillin G, succinylcholine, vancomycin.

Nursing Considerations

- Use 4.2% solution for IV administration. Dilute 8.4% solution 1:1 with compatible dilute for IV administration.
- Infuse slowly IV push over 5–10 minutes ($\leq$1 mEq/minute).
- Flush IV before and after drug administration if IV solution contains calcium or magnesium.
- Use large vein for administration.
- Observe IV site closely for extravasation.
- Monitor vital signs.
- Monitor serum electrolytes, calcium, osmolality, blood pH, CO_2, and base deficit.
- Administer PO with feeding to decrease GI irritation. Dilute with some formula or breast milk.
- Observe for signs of gastric irritation: vomiting, gastric residuals, diarrhea, abdominal distention, gastric residuals or stools positive for occult blood.
- Monitor kidney function.
- Observe for signs of excessive alkalosis (hyperirritability, respiratory depression, and seizures).
- Do not use if discolored or contains precipitate.
- Sodium content: 12 mEq/gm (1 mEq HCO_3^- = 1 mEq Na^+).
- Osmolality (injection 1 mEq/ml): 1555 mOsm/kg H_2O.

Sodium Chloride

Brand Names

Various

Forms

Injection 2.5 mEq/ml and 4 mEq/ml.

Uses

Prevention and treatment of hyponatremia (serum sodium <130–135 mEq/L).

Dose

2–4 mEq/kg/day in IV continuous infusion or PO in 2–4 divided doses. Higher doses may be needed during the first weeks of life. Adjust dose as indicated by serum sodium. Dose is total intake, including PO feedings.

Pharmacokinetics

Well absorbed from the GI tract after PO administration. Excreted mainly by the kidneys. Losses are increased with vomiting and diarrhea.

Cautions

Large doses or rapid IV administration can cause hypernatremia, hypervolemia, and pulmonary and brain edema. Large doses of chloride may cause a loss of bicarbonate resulting in metabolic acidosis. Hypernatremia (>150 mEq/L) can cause irritability, tremors, and seizures. Hyperosmolar. Intravenous administration can cause phlebitis. Gastrointestinal irritation can occur with PO administration.

Use with caution in infants with heart failure or severe kidney dysfunction and in infants receiving steroids.

Solution Compatibility

Compatible with most IV solutions, including TPN and fat emulsion 10%.

Additive Compatibility

Compatible with most drugs.

Nursing Considerations

- Administer IV by continuous infusion.
- Administer PO with feeding to decrease GI irritation. Dilute with some formula or breast milk.
- Observe for signs of gastric irritation: vomiting, gastric residuals, diarrhea, abdominal distention, gastric residuals or stools positive for occult blood.
- Monitor serum sodium, chloride, and osmolality (ask yourself: is hyponatremia or hypernatremia due to increased or decreased extracellular fluid).
- Monitor I and O and kidney function.
- Observe/monitor for signs of dehydration: tachycardia, hypotension, depressed fontanelle, dry mucous membranes, poor skin turgor, decreased urine output (<2 ml/kg/hour), increased urine specific gravity, and metabolic acidosis.
- Observe/monitor for signs of fluid overload: increased respiratory distress, rales, peripheral edema, and marked increase in weight.
- Observe for signs of HYPOnatremia: hyperactivity and seizures (hyponatremia is usually asymptomatic when due to chronic rather than acute development). Changes in EKG include: increased duration and amplitude of QRS complex, shortened QT_c interval, and inverted ST and T waves.

Vitamins, Minerals, and Electrolytes   **231**

- Observe for signs of HYPERnatremia: irritability, tremors, seizures, oliguria, and apnea. Changes in EKG include: decreased duration and amplitude of QRS complex and lengthened QT_c interval.
- Osmolality (injection 2.5 mEq/ml): 5370 mOsm/kg H_2O (FP).

Chapter 10

Vaccines and Toxoids

Diphtheria and Tetanus Toxoids and Pertussis Vaccine Adsorbed (DTP)

Brand Names

Tri-Immunol, various

Forms

Injection 0.5 ml (diphtheria toxoid 12.5 Lf units, tetanus toxoid 5 Lf units, and pertussis vaccine ~4 protective units) in 5 ml and 7.5 ml vials (for IM use).

Uses

Provides active immunity to diphtheria, tetanus, and pertussis in infants and children 6 weeks through 6 years of age.

Dose

0.5 ml at 2 months, 4 months, 6 months, and between 15 and 18 months of age. A single dose does not provide protection against diphtheria, tetanus, or pertussis.
Preterm infants should receive primary immunizations with the usual dose at the usual chronologic ages.

Pharmacokinetics

Immunity to diphtheria and tetanus persists for at least 10 years in most children following primary immunization with four doses of DTP. Immunity to pertussis begins to decrease between 4 and 6 years following primary immunization.

Cautions

Can cause mild to moderate fever (>38°C), chills, vomiting, irritability, poor appetite, and malaise within 3–6 hours after administration, persisting for 1–2 days. Local reaction can cause tenderness, swelling, erythema, and induration at the injection site. A nodule may be palpable at the injection site for a few weeks. Contraindicated in infants with an active infection. Rarely, a serious reaction (presumably caused by the pertussis component) can cause fever (>39°C), irritability, screaming (for long periods), excessive sleepiness, seizures, and shock.

Pertussis vaccine is CONTRAINDICATED in infants with a history of seizures or previous serious reaction to DTP.

Drug Interactions

Corticosteroids: concurrent use of corticosteriods may decrease efficacy of vaccine or toxoid.

Nursing Considerations

• Do NOT administer DTP to infants with history of seizures or previous serious reaction to DTP. Use

DT (diphtheria and tetanus toxoid adsorbed, for pediatric use) ONLY.
- Use anterolateral thigh for IM administration to infants.
- Shake container of DTP vigorously prior to withdrawing dose.
- Do not use if clumps are seen after vigorous shaking or if resuspension cannot be achieved.
- Monitor infant's temperature. Consider prophylactic use of acetaminophen to minimize fever and irritability.
- Refrigerate.
- Record date of administration, manufacturer, lot number and name, address and title of person administering vaccine in infant's permanent medical record (required by the National Childhood Vaccine Injury Act).
- Initiate official immunization record for infant. Give immunization record to parents on infant's discharge from the hospital.

Hepatitis B Virus Vaccine Inactivated (Plasma-derived)

Brand Names

Heptavax-B (pediatric formulation)

Forms

Injection 10 mcg (of hepatitis B surface antigen) in 0.5 ml vials (for IM use).

Uses

Postexposure prophylaxis in neonates born to mothers who are hepatitis B surface antigen (HBsAg) positive. Provides active immunity.
Used in conjunction with hepatitis B immune globulin.

Dose

10 mcg (0.5 ml) IM at birth.
Repeat dose at 1 and 6 months of age.

Pharmacokinetics

Anti-HBs appear in the serum within 2 weeks after administration, peaks at 6 months, and persists for at least 3 years.

Cautions

Can cause a slight fever and infrequently, rash, vomiting, diarrhea, abdominal pain, lethargy, and poor appetite. Local reaction can cause pain, swelling, warmth, and induration at the injection site, which usually subsides within 2 days.

Contraindicated in neonates and infants with a serious, active infection or severely compromised cardiopulmonary status.

Drug Interactions

Corticosteroids: concurrent use of corticosteroids may decrease efficacy of vaccine or toxoid.

Nursing Considerations

* Use anterolateral thigh for IM administration.
* Administer as soon as possible after birth (within 7 days).

- Administer first dose of hepatitis B virus vaccine inactivated with hepatitis B immune globulin at separate sites.
- Monitor infant's temperature.
- Test infant for the presence of anti-HBsAg at 9–12 months of age.
- Refrigerate.

NOTE If HBsAg positive mother is identified >1 month after giving birth, the infant should be screened for HBsAg. If the infant tests negative, administer one dose of hepatitis immune globulin (immediately) and three doses of hepatitis B virus vaccine inactivated (immediately and at 1 and 6 months of age).

Poliovirus Vaccines: Live Oral Trivalent (OPV) and Inactivated (IPV)

Brand Names

Orimune Trivalent (OPV) for PO use.
Poliovirus Vaccine Inactivated (IPV) for SQ use only.

Forms

Oral solution 0.5 ml single dose disposable pipettes (Dispettes).
Injection 1 ml ampuls, 10 ml vials.

Uses

Provide active immunity to poliomyelitis caused by poliovirus types 1, 2, and 3. In the U.S. OPV is the vaccine of choice for primary immunization in immunocompetent infants and children 6 weeks through 17 years of age. For immunocompromised (immunodeficient or immunosuppressed) infants and children, IPV is the vaccine of choice.

Dose

OPV 0.5 ml PO or IPV 1 ml SQ at 2 months, 4 months, and between 15 and 18 months of age (primary OPV or IPV immunization is commonly integrated with DTP immunizations).
Preterm infants should receive primary immunizations with the usual dose at the usual chronologic ages.

Pharmacokinetics

Duration of immunity to the poliovirus following primary immunization with OPV or currently available IPV has not been established. Vaccine viruses are shed in nasal secretions, saliva, urine, and stools for at least 6–8 weeks after administration.

Cautions

Rarely, paralytic poliomyelitis has occurred after administration of OPV, with an increased risk in vaccine recipients who are immunocompromised. Nonimmune and immunocompromised close personal contacts are also at risk for OPV-associated disease. Erythema and tenderness at injection site, fever ($\geq$38.5°C) on day of vaccination and persisting for 1–2 days, and sensitivity with urticarial rash or anaphylaxis can occur after administration of IPV. Both OPV and IPV are contraindicated in infants with acute illnesses.
   OPV is CONTRAINDICATED in infants with immuno-

deficiency diseases and infants with hypogammaglobulinemia or agammaglobulinemia.

Drug Interactions

Corticosteroids: concurrent use of corticosteroids may decrease efficacy of vaccine or toxoid.

Nursing Considerations

- To avoid cross infection, do NOT administer OPV while infant is still in the hospital. Initiate OPV immunization on infant's discharge from the hospital.
- Do NOT administer OPV to immunocompromised infants.
- Can administer OPV with water or formula.
- Administer IPV via SQ injection ONLY (preferably into tissue near the insertion of the deltoid muscle).
- Monitor infant's temperature after IPV administration.
- Instruct nonimmune or immunocompromised close contacts regarding shedding of virus in nasal and oral secretions, urine, and stools.
- OPV is clear, red to pink to yellow in color. Keep frozen until just prior to use.
- IPV is clear, pink to red in color. Refrigerate. Do not freeze.
- Record date of administration, manufacturer, lot number and name, address and title of person administering vaccine in infant's permanent medical record (required by the National Childhood Vaccine Injury Act).
- Initiate official immunization record for infant. Give immunization record to parents on infant's discharge from the hospital.

NOTE Administration of OPV or IPV to infants <6 weeks of age is not generally recommended because most infants have maternal antibodies that may prevent a satisfactory immunologic response to the virus vaccine; however, OPV or IPV should be administered if the infant is traveling to a country where poliomyelitis is endemic.

Chapter 11

Miscellaneous Drugs

Normal Serum Albumin, Human 5% and 25%

Brand Names

Albuminar-5, Plasbumin-5, various
Albuminar-25, Plasbumin-25, various

Forms

50 mg/ml in 50 ml and 250 ml bottles (5%).
1 gm/4 ml in 20 ml, 50 ml, and 100 ml bottles (25%).

Contents

Contains no less than 96% of the total protein as albumin, no clotting factors.

Uses

Volume expansion.
Replacement of plasma loss due to conditions such as capillary leak syndrome (sepsis) or sequestration of protein-rich fluids (peritonitis).
Treatment of hypoproteinemia with edema in the pre-term infant.
Adjunct to exchange transfusion in the treatment of hyperbilirubinemia.

Dose

Replacement of plasma loss/volume expansion 5–10 ml/kg IV infusion (5%) prn.
Treatment of hypoproteinemia 4 ml (1 gm)/kg IV infusion (25%) prn.
Adjunct to exchange transfusion 4 ml (1 gm)/kg IV infusion (25%), 1–2 hours prior to exchange transfusion.

Cautions

Can cause fever, vomiting, and urticarial rash. Can also cause fluid overload, especially with rapid administration. Administration of large quantities can cause relative anemia.

Use with caution in infants with kidney dysfunction and in asphyxiated infants. Contraindicated in infants with severe anemia or heart failure.

Nursing Considerations

- Use filter supplied by manufacturer or 150-μm blood filter.
- Infuse slowly IV over 30 minutes–2 hours, as tolerated.
- Monitor fluid status: HR, RR, BP, acid-base balance, and urine output.
- Observe/monitor for signs of hypovolemia: tachycardia, metabolic acidosis, decreased urine output (<1–2 ml/kg/hour).
- Observe/monitor for signs of acute fluid overload: increased respiratory distress, rales, increased pCO_2, decreased pO_2 or O_2 saturation.
- Monitor total serum protein.

- Monitor hematocrit/hemoglobin.
- May dilute 25% solution to 5% by mixing 16 ml D5W or 0.9% NaCl with 4 ml of 25% solution.
- Use product within 4 hours after opening.
- Do not use if solution is turbid or contains precipitate.
- Sodium content: 13 mEq/100 ml.

Heparin

Brand Names

Liquamin, various

Forms

Injection 1,000 units/ml, 5,000 units/ml, 10,000 units/ml (may contain benzyl alcohol or other preservatives). Heparin lock flush 10 units/ml, 100 units/ml (may contain benzyl alcohol or other preservatives).

Uses

Anticoagulant. Used to maintain patency of central venous and arterial catheters and peripheral "lock" catheters (used for intermittent injection of drugs and solutions) by preventing clot formation.

Dose

0.5–2 units/ml for continuous parenteral solutions. 10 units/ml for peripheral "lock" catheters. Infuse JUST enough to flush tip of catheter q 4–6 hours prn.

Pharmacokinetics

Rapid onset of action (within minutes) after IV administration. Highly bound to plasma proteins and fibrinogen in the blood; therefore, distribution is limited. Metabolic fate is not fully defined. Taken up by reticuloendothelial cells. May be partially metabolized in the liver with small amounts of heparin eliminated unchanged in the urine. Half-life is 1–2 hours. A major change in urine output may alter heparin clearance and its duration of activity.

Cautions

The major adverse effect is, of course, bleeding. Serious bleeding is very rare with doses of 1 unit/ml in parenteral fluids. Protamine is used to reverse the effects of overheparinization (1 mg protamine neutralizes 100 units of heparin; see "Protamine" review). Use may also cause mild, reversible thrombocytopenia, increased SGOT and SGPT (without increases in bilirubin and alkaline phosphatase), and hypersensitivity reactions with fever, rash, asthma-like symptoms, and vomiting.

Heparin flush solutions MUST be nonpreserved. The major source of benzyl alcohol identified by Gershanik et al. and Brown et al. in infants with "Gasping syndrome" was saline and heparin flushes preserved with benzyl alcohol.

Heparinization is CONTRAINDICATED in infants with a history of a recent bleeding episode (intracranial or GI hemorrhage). Thrombocytopenia is a relative contraindication to heparin therapy.

Solution Compatibility

D5W, D10W, 0.9% NaCl, TPN.

Additive Compatibility

Aminophylline, amphotericin B, ampicillin, calcium gluconate, chloramphenicol, cimetidine, clindamycin, dobutamine (at low heparin concentrations), dopamine, gentamicin (at concentrations of 1 unit/ml or less), hydrocortisone, isoproterenol, methicillin, methylprednisolone, metronidazole (with sodium bicarbonate), nafcillin, penicillin G, potassium chloride, sodium bicarbonate.

Additive Incompatibility

Amikacin (at concentrations greater than 1 unit/ml), hyaluronidase, meperidine, morphine, tobramycin, vancomycin.

Nursing Considerations

- Observe infant for signs of bleeding (note bruising, check gastric residuals and stools for occult blood, monitor hematocrit/hemoglobin).
- Monitor platelet count.
- Monitor liver and kidney function.
- Heparin infusions may reduce serum triglyceride levels in infants receiving IV fat emulsion (e.g., Intralipid).
- Use ONLY nonpreserved, single-use, heparin lock flush solutions.

NOTE In the interest of safety, and for ease of calculation, stock heparin in a neonatal intensive care unit should be confined to one concentration for parenteral infusions (e.g., 1000 units/ml) and one concentration for lock flush (10 units/ml nonpreserved).

Miscellaneous Drugs   **245**

Hepatitis B Immune Globulin

Brand Names

H-BIG, various

Forms

Injection 0.5 ml in 1 ml, 4 ml, and 5 ml vials or 0.5 ml syringe (for IM use).

Uses

Postexposure prophylaxis in neonates born to mothers who are hepatitis B surface antigen (HBsAg) positive. Provides passive immunity.
Used in conjunction with hepatitis B virus vaccine inactivated.

Dose

0.5 ml IM (one dose) at birth.

Pharmacokinetics

Anti-HBs appears in the serum between 1 and 6 days after administration, peaks at 3–11 days, and persists for 2–6 months.

Cautions

Can cause rash, fever, lethargy, and rarely anaphylaxis. Intravenous administration can cause a serious allergic reaction. Local reaction can cause pain, tenderness, swelling, and erythema at the injection site.

Nursing Considerations

- Use anterolateral thigh for IM administration.
- Do NOT administer IV.

- Administer as soon as possible after birth (within 12 hours). Delayed administration results in progressive loss of efficacy.
- Administer hepatitis B immune globulin with hepatitis B virus vaccine inactivated at separate sites.
- Monitor infant's temperature.
- Test infant for presence of anti-HBsAg at 9–12 months of age.
- Refrigerate.

NOTE If HBsAg positive mother is identified >1 month after giving birth, the infant should be screened for HBsAg. If the infant tests negative, administer one dose of hepatitis immune globulin (immediately) and three doses of hepatitis B virus vaccine inactivated (immediately and at 1 and 6 months of age).

Hyaluronidase

Brand Name

Wydase

Forms

Injection 150 units (for reconstitution).

Uses

Reduces dermal necrosis and sloughing after IV extravasation of calcium, nafcillin, or other "toxic" infiltrates (enhances absorption and dispersion of drug).

Dose

150 unit vial reconstituted with 1 ml of 0.9% NaCl. Intradermal.

Use tuberculin syringe with 25 gauge needle,
infiltrate in 0.1 ml volumes throughout the affected
area.

Cautions

Occasional sensitivity reaction with rash occurs.

Nursing Considerations

- Administer drug ASAP after extravasation.
- Do NOT administer IV.
- Gently cleanse skin with povidone-iodine or alcohol
  prior to infiltration of drug throughout affected area.
- Document appearance of lesion prior to administra-
  tion (size, color, presence of swelling, induration,
  blanching or blister).
- Consider plastic surgery consultation.
- Do not use if discolored or contains precipitate
  (drug may normally appear hazy).

Immune Serum Globulin, Human (IV)

Brand Names

Sandoglobulin, Gamimune (with maltose 10%), various

Forms

Injection 1 gm, 3 gm, 6 gm (for reconstitution to 3% or
6% concentration).
Injection 50 mg/ml in 10 ml, 50 ml, and 100 ml vials
(5% concentration).

Contents

Contain 96% IgG and traces of IgA and IgM.

Uses

Used to reduce incidence, or morbidity and mortality of septicemia in VLBW infants (<1500 gm, <32–34 weeks' gestation).
Provides passive immunity.

Dose

Prophylaxis: 500 mg/kg q week.
Septicemia: 500 mg/kg q day for 3–6 days.
Monitor serum IgG levels. Minimum effective dose and optimal duration of therapy not established.

Pharmacokinetics

Appears in the serum immediately after IV infusion.
Half-life is ~11 days in the preterm infant to 20–30 days in the term infant.

Cautions

Can cause vomiting, fever, rash, flushing, respiratory distress, and rarely, a precipitous fall in BP and anaphylaxis. These effects are usually related to the rate of infusion.

Solution Compatibility

D5W.

Additive Compatibility

Do NOT mix with other drugs.

Nursing Considerations

- Administer immediately after reconstitution.
- Infuse slowly IV over 4–6 hours.

- Use a controlled infusion device for administration.
- Monitor HR, RR, temperature, and BP during infusion. Obtain baseline values prior to initiation of infusion.
- Stop or decrease infusion if undesired effects occur (until undesired effects subside). Resume infusion at a slower rate.
- Monitor serum IgG level.
  Most placental transfer of IgG occurs after the 32nd–34th week of gestation, increasing throughout gestation. Levels are low at birth in the preterm infant (<400–600 mg/dl) and do not increase appreciably until about 15 weeks of age.
- Refrigerate.

Phentolamine

Brand Name

Regitine

Forms

Injection 5 mg (for reconstitution).

Use

Prevents dermal necrosis and sloughing after IV extravasation of epinephrine or dopamine.

Dose

5 mg vial reconstituted with 10 ml of 0.9% NaCl.
Intradermal.
Use tuberculin syringe with 25 gauge needle, infiltrate in 0.1 ml volumes throughout the affected area.

Cautions

Intravenous administration can cause hypotension, tachycardia, arrhythmias, vomiting, and diarrhea.

Nursing Considerations

- Administer drug ASAP after extravasation. Effective only if administered within 12 hours after extravasation.
- Do NOT administer IV.
- Expect hyperemia at site after infiltration of phentolamine.
- Gently cleanse skin with povidone-iodine or alcohol prior to infiltration of drug throughout affected area.
- Document appearance of lesion prior to administration (size, color, presence of swelling, induration, blanching or blister).
- Consider plastic surgery consultation.

Protamine

Brand Names

Various

Forms

Injection 10 mg/ml in 5 ml ampuls and 25 ml vials, and in 50 mg and 250 mg vials for reconstitution (may contain preservatives).

Uses

Heparin antagonist. Used to reverse SEVERE bleeding due to heparin overdose.

Dose

1 mg protamine neutralizes approximately 100 units of heparin.

Administer 1 mg for every 100 units of heparin estimated to remain in infant (advantageous to slightly underestimate protamine dose; see "Cautions").

Pharmacokinetics

Rapid onset of action. Neutralizing of heparin occurs within 5 minutes after IV administration. Metabolic fate is unknown. The protamine-heparin complex has no activity as an anticoagulant.

Cautions

Protamine has weak anticoagulant activity when not complexed with heparin. Overestimation of the amount of heparin remaining in infant may result in an excess of protamine exerting its own anticoagulant activity and causing bleeding. Hypotension, bradycardia, dyspnea, transient flushing and hypersensitivity reactions with rash, pulmonary edema, and anaphylaxis can occur with use.

First, DISCONTINUE heparin infusion. Then attempt to calculate amount of heparin remaining in infant. Heparin has a short-life (60 minutes). If bleeding is not severe or the time elapsed since a heparin bolus was infused is >2 hours, protamine may not be indicated. Reduce protamine dose by 50% if time elapsed is 30–60 minutes, and reduce protamine dose by 75% if time elapsed is ≥2 hours. The majority of heparin overdoses can be managed by simply discontinuing the heparin infusion and monitoring coagulation times.

Solution Compatibility

D5W, 0.9% NaCl.

Additive Compatibility

Do NOT mix with other drugs.

Nursing Considerations

- Infuse slowly IV over 3–5 minutes (maximum rate 5 mg/minute).
- Monitor HR, respiratory effort, and BP.
- Observe infant for continued bleeding.
- Monitor coagulation studies (PTT or ACT). Obtain 5–15 minutes after drug administration and at 2–8 hours if indicated.
- Refrigerate drug.

Sodium Polystyrene Sulfonate

Brand Names

Kayexalate, various

Forms

Powder, for suspension.
Suspension 1.25 gm/5 ml (contains alcohol, preservatives, and sorbitol 33%).

Uses

Treatment of hyperkalemia (>6.5 mEq/L). Used alone if no cardiac symptoms or concomitantly with other measures (sodium bicarbonate, calcium, or insulin and glucose) if cardiac symptoms present.

Dose

0.5–1 gm/kg/dose PO, PR q 4–6 hours prn.

Pharmacokinetics

Onset of action is within 1–2 hours (PR > PO). Duration of effect is 4–6 hours. Conversion of resin to potassium form occurs principally in the large intestine due to the high concentration of potassium present. One gram of resin (drug) releases 1 mEq of sodium in exchange for 1 mEq of potassium. The modified resin is excreted in the feces.

Cautions

Overtreatment can result in hypokalemia and possibly hypernatremia. Cation exchange is not selective for potassium and can include calcium and magnesium, resulting in hypocalcemia or hypomagnesemia. Can cause gastric irritation and vomiting (PO administration) and constipation (oral and rectal route). Sorbitol is used as laxative to avoid constipation and bezoar formation which can result in intestinal obstruction and possible hemorrhage.

Use with caution in digitalized infants and in infants with heart failure.

Drug Interactions

Antacids: concurrent PO administration may reduce the resin's potassium exchanging capacity. Concurrent PO administration of magnesium-containing antacid may result in metabolic alkalosis in infants with kidney failure.

Nursing Considerations

- STOP all potassium administration.
- See "Potassium Chloride: Nursing Considerations," for treatment of hyperkalemia with cardiac symptoms.
- Shake suspension well before drawing up dose.
- Administer PO by orogastric or nasogastric feeding tube. Do not administer with feeding.
- Administer slowly PR by lubricated feeding tube. Hold or secure buttocks together after administration for optimal retention (for at least 15 minutes).
- Do not heat suspension (changes in the exchange properties of the resin may occur).
- Observe for signs of gastric irritation, constipation, and intestinal obstruction: increased abdominal girth, visible loops of bowel, vomiting, gastric residuals or stools positive for occult or gross blood.
- Monitor serum electrolytes, calcium, and magnesium.
- Monitor EKG.
- Observe for signs of HYPOkalemia: drowsiness, hypotonia, poor feeding, and tachycardia. Changes in EKG include: prolonged QT_c interval, depressed ST segment, flat or inverted T wave, appearance of U wave, prolonged PR interval, prominent P wave, and ectopic beats (supraventricular and ventricular). Digoxin (toxic) effects enhanced in hypokalemia.
- Observe for signs of HYPERkalemia: hypotonia, cold skin, gray pallor, hypotension, cardiac arrhythmias, heart block, and possible asystole. Changes in EKG include: tall, peaked T waves (earliest mani-

festation), widening of QRS complex, PR and QT_c
intervals, wide and flattened P waves, ectopic
rhythms, and heart block. Effects are enhanced by
hyponatremia, hypocalcemia, or acidosis.
- Store at room temperature.
- Sodium content: 1 mEq/ml of available suspension.
  4.1 mEq/gm of powder resin.

Tromethamine

Brand Name

THAM (tris-hydroxymethyl-aminomethane)

Forms

Injection 500 ml bottle of 0.3M solution.

Uses

Alkalinizing agent. Correction of documented
metabolic acidosis without increasing serum sodium
or carbon dioxide.

Dose

1 mEq (3.3 ml of 0.3M solution)/kg/dose IV.
Doses should be based on pH and base deficit:

$$\text{dose (ml of 0.3M THAM)} = \text{weight (kg)} \times 1.1 \times \text{base deficit (mEq/ml)}$$

Maximum dose is 40 ml/kg (~12 mEq/kg) over 24
hours.

Pharmacokinetics

Rapidly excreted in the urine with no appreciable
metabolism.

Cautions

Can cause respiratory depression and apnea, transient hypoglycemia or hyperglycemia, hyperkalemia, and osmotic diuresis.

Contraindicated in infants with kidney failure.

Solution Compatibility

D5W.

Additive Compatibility

Do NOT mix with other drugs.

Nursing Considerations

- Infuse slowly IV push over 2–5 minute (≤1 ml/minute).
- Monitor blood gases (pH, pCO_2, pO_2, base deficit).
- Monitor kidney function and urine output.
- Monitor blood glucose and serum potassium.
- Observe for signs of excessive alkalosis (hyperirritability, respiratory depression, and seizures).

Urokinase

Brand Names

Abbokinase, Open-cath

Forms

5000 unit vials (for reconstitution).

Uses

Used to restore patency of occluded central catheters by promoting thrombolysis.

Dose

Reconstitute vial with nonpreserved sterile water for injection to provide solution containing 5000 units/ml. Using sterile technique, disconnect IV tubing from occluded catheter and attach a 1 ml syringe, containing drug solution, to the catheter. Slowly inject enough urokinase volume to JUST fill the catheter. Replace urokinase syringe with empty 6 ml syringe. Allow urokinase to remain in catheter for 5 minutes, then attempt to gently aspirate enough volume to remove all urokinase solution, any remaining clot, and 4–5 ml of blood into the 6 ml syringe. Repeat attempts to aspirate every 5 minutes until catheter is successfully cleared. May repeat entire procedure after 30 minutes. After catheter is successfully cleared, flush catheter with 0.9% NaCl, and aseptically replace IV tubing.

Cautions

Though there are no adverse effects reported when drug is used for removal of clots occluding central catheters, possible reactions should be considered. The major adverse effect is bleeding (superficial and internal). Do NOT inject any urokinase solution into the infant. The volume of urokinase solution injected into the catheter should be sufficient to just fill JUST the catheter. Be sure to aspirate enough volume to remove all urokinase, any remaining clot, and 4–5 ml blood. Use can also cause hypersensitivity reactions with bronchospasm, rash, and fever.

Drug Interactions

Anticoagulants: increased chance of bleeding possible when urokinase used in infants receiving heparin.

Indomethacin: drugs reducing platelet function, such as indomethacin, may increase risk of bleeding when used concurrently with urokinase.

Additive Compatibility

Do NOT mix with other drugs.

Nursing Considerations

- Inject JUST enough urokinase solution SLOWLY and GENTLY to fill catheter. Excessive force may dislodge clot into circulation.
- Take care NOT to inject urokinase into infant.
- Observe infant for signs of superficial bleeding (IV sites, puncture sites, and fresh surgical wounds) and internal bleeding (GI hemorrhage and IVH).
- Monitor hematocrit/hemoglobin.
- Monitor infant's temperature.
- Observe infant for wheezing and rash.
- Drug is not effective in restoring patency of catheters occluded by drug precipitates.
- Refrigerate powder and reconstituted solution.

Appendices

Appendix A

Cardiopulmonary Resuscitation

Resuscitation is required more often in the first few minutes of life than at any other time, though infants may require resuscitation any time that ventilation or circulation is ineffective. Circulatory failure and/or arrest is usually the result of profound hypoxemia and acidosis from respiratory failure and/or arrest or shock and is rarely due to primary cardiac dysfunction. The "ABC's" of CPR must be carried out by personnel skillful in neonatal/infant resuscitation and capable of functioning as a team.

Airway

Proper alignment and patency of the airway is essential.
- Place infant on its back or left side with neck in a neutral position.
- Place a 1-inch-thick roll under the shoulders to maintain proper airway position.
- Avoid overextension or underextension of the neck, which may cause airway obstruction.
- GENTLY suction first the nose, then the mouth.
- Avoid vigorous and deep suctioning of the oropharynx which may cause vagal stimulation with bradycardia and/or apnea.

Breathing

If spontaneous respirations are absent or ineffective, assisted ventilation should be initiated.

- Initiate assisted ventilation at 40 breaths/minute with a bag and mask.
- If unable to inflate lungs, reposition airway and face mask.
- Intubate if inadequate ventilation after 15–30 seconds with a bag and mask.
- Signs of adequate ventilation include:
  - bilateral chest expansion.
  - auscultation of breath sounds.
  - increased HR.
  - improved color and peripheral pulses.
- Avoid vigorous ventilation, which can produce barotrauma and pulmonary air leaks. Ventilate with just enough pressure to move the chest.
- Assess the HR after 15–30 seconds of adequate ventilation.
- Discontinue assisted ventilation if HR > 100 and effective spontaneous respirations are present.

Circulation

External chest compressions should be initiated if HR is <60/minute or <80/minute and not increasing with 100% oxygen and ADEQUATE ventilation for 30 seconds.

- Initiate external chest compressions at a rate of 120 compressions/minute.
- Place your thumbs over the middle third of the sternum, just below the nipple line, and encircle the infant's torso with your fingers to support its back (superimpose thumbs for compression of the very

small infant), **or** place your ring or index and middle fingers on the sternum, one finger breadth below the nipple line, and use your other hand to support the infant's back.

- Compress the sternum ½–¾ inch.
- Do NOT compress the lower portion of the sternum because of potential damage to abdominal organs.
- Check brachial and femoral pulses and BP to assess effectiveness of compressions.
- Accompany chest compressions with assisted ventilation at 40–60 breaths/minute. There are no current recommendations for coordination of ventilation and chest compressions.
- Assess HR after 30 seconds of chest compressions.
- Discontinue chest compressions when spontaneous HR ≥ 80/minute.

Drugs

Drugs should be administered if, after ADEQUATE ventilation with 100% oxygen and chest compressions, the HR remains <80/minute. Oxygen, epinephrine, naloxone, and volume expanders are the drugs of choice for NEONATAL resuscitation.

- **Epinephrine** 0.01–0.03 mg/kg (0.1–0.3 ml/kg 1 : 10,000 solution) IV, ET, IC q 5 minutes prn is indicated for the treatment of asystole or a HR < 80 despite adequate ventilation with 100% oxygen and chest compressions.
- **Naloxone** 0.01 mg/kg of a neonatal solution (0.02 mg/ml) IV, ET q 2–3 minutes prn is indicated for the reversal of narcotic-induced respiratory depression.
- **Volume expansion** (with crystalloid or colloid) 10 ml/kg is indicated in the presence of hypovolemia.

Suspect hypovolemia if pallor, weak peripheral pulses, hypotension, and poor capillary refill persist despite adequate ventilation, oxygenation, and spontaneous HR > 100.

Atropine, calcium, and sodium bicarbonate are no longer recommended in the acute phase of NEONATAL resuscitation. Calcium is indicated ONLY for the treatment of DOCUMENTED hypocalcemia or hyperkalemia with cardiotoxicity. Sodium bicarbonate is indicated ONLY for the treatment of DOCUMENTED metabolic acidosis during prolonged resuscitation. Drugs to improve cardiac output and BP (e.g., dopamine, dobutamine) and drugs to control heart rhythm and rate (e.g., atropine, isoproterenol, lidocaine) may be indicated for the resuscitation and stabilization of the older neonate and infant with significant pulmonary and/or cardiac disease.

Ideally drugs should be administered IV during resuscitation, but when venous access is not readily available, the ETT is the most easily accessible route for the delivery of epinepherine and naloxone ONLY. The epinepherine or naloxone dose may be diluted 1:1 with NS to aid in the delivery via the ETT. Intramuscular and SQ routes have little value in resuscitation due to slow and unpredictable absorption of drugs. Intracardiac route should be used ONLY in infants without ET or IV access. Intracardiac drug administration may cause pneumothorax, hemopericardium, coronary artery laceration, myocardial necrosis (with injection of drug into the myocardium), and irreversible arrhythmias.

Every high-risk neonate and infant should have individualized resuscitation information at their bedside. This information should include the ETT size and drug and cardioversion/defibrillation doses appropriate for infant's weight. This information should be updated periodically with growth of the infant.

Nursing Considerations During Resuscitation

- Note time resuscitation attempt began.
- Remove unnecessary people.
- Assist in the "ABC's" of CPR.
- Provide warm environment for infant.
- Assess heart tones, breath sounds, and peripheral pulses at intervals.
- Monitor HR, rhythm, BP, and temperature.
- Monitor blood gases, glucose, hematocrit, electrolytes, and calcium.
- Assist with chest radiograph and/or transillumination of chest.

Nursing Considerations Postresuscitation

- Document all observations and actions in infant's chart.
- Obtain blood gas, glucose, hematocrit, electrolytes, and calcium.
- Monitor HR, rhythm, BP, respiratory effort, and temperature.
- Resolve problems encountered during resuscitation (e.g., equipment malfunction, unavailable drugs, etc.).
- Assure that parents have been notified of "event."

Appendix B

Electrocardiogram

A 12-lead ECG allows for the assessment of heart rhythm and chamber function. It consists of six limb leads and six chest leads. In a normally positioned heart, leads V_1–V_3 provide information about the right heart, and V_4–V_6 provide information about the left heart.

Placement of Leads

Limb leads include bipolar leads I (R arm/L arm), II (R arm/L leg), and III (L arm/L leg) and unipolar leads aV_R (R arm), aV_L (L arm), and aV_F (L leg).

Chest leads include: V_1 4th R intercostal space at R sternal border

V_2 4th L intercostal space at L sternal border

V_3 halfway between V_2 and V_4

V_4 5th L intercostal space at L midclavicular line

V_5 5th L intercostal space at L anterior axillary line

V_6 5th L intercostal space at L mid axillary line

V_7 5th L intercostal space at L

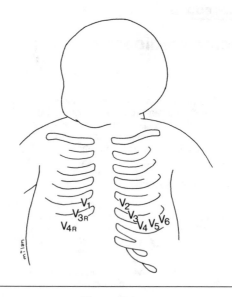

Figure B.1.

posterior axillary line (used if there is no Q wave in V_6)

V_{3R} V_3 on R chest (used in place of V_3 in infants)

V_{4R} V_4 on R chest

Figure B.1 indicates placement of chest leads.

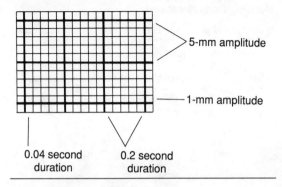

Figure B.2.

Interpretation of ECG

To interpret an ECG, it is necessary to measure amplitude and duration of complexes. At a speed of 25 mm/second, each of the smallest squares of paper is equal to 0.04 seconds duration horizontally and 1 mm amplitude vertically; each larger square is equal to 0.2 seconds duration and 5 mm amplitude (Fig. B.2).

Normal ECG Values

PR Interval   0.07–0.14 seconds (varies with age
                             and HR)
QRS Duration 0.04–0.08 seconds (varies with age)
QT_c Interval   0.4–0.44 seconds (corrected for HR)
Normal values for amplitudes will vary with the infant's age and the lead used.

Nursing Considerations

- Set speed at 25 mm/second (use 50 mm/second if a more accurate and clear reading is indicated).
- Keep infant as quiet as possible.
- Expose infant's chest. Provide a warm environment.
- Do NOT use alcohol pads for conduction; serious burns can result.
- Cleanse infant's skin of conduction cream or paste after completion of ECG.

Appendix C

Cardioversion and Defibrillation

Synchronized Cardioversion

Used to convert paroxysmal atrial tachycardia (PAT), atrial flutter, atrial fibrillation, and rarely supraventricular tachycardia (SVT) unresponsive to antiarrhythmic drugs, in infants who are symptomatic with poor perfusion, hypotension, and heart failure. Used to restore normal sinus rhythm. For cardioversion, the SYNCHRONIZER mode MUST be used. Use of the defibrillator mode may induce ventricular fibrillation.

Dose

0.2–1 W-sec (joules)/kg. Begin at the lowest dose and increase with subsequent attempts.

Correct hypoxemia, acidosis, hypoglycemia, and hypothermia if present.

Caution

CONTRAINDICATED in infants with arrhythmias caused by digoxin toxicity.

Doses ≥5 W-sec/kg can cause severe myocardial burns, congestive cardiomyopathy, decreased contractility, and death.

Defibrillation

Used to convert ventricular fibrillation and rarely ventricular tachycardia ONLY. Used to restore normal sinus rhythm.

For defibrillation, the defibrillator mode is used.

Dose

2 W-sec (joules)/kg. If unsuccessful, the energy dose should be doubled.

Correct hypoxemia, acidosis, hypoglycemia, and hypothermia if present.

Administration of epinephrine or lidocaine may facilitate defibrillation.,

Caution

Doses $\geq$5 W-sec/kg can cause severe myocardial burns, congestive cardiomyopathy, decreased contractility, and death.

Procedure for Cardioversion or Defibrillation

- Consider administration of analgesic to infant prior to elective cardioversion.
- Maintain infant on dry surface. Provide warm environment.
- Use appropriate size paddles (4.5 cm recommended for infants). Internal adult paddles are often used.
- Use electrode cream or paste or saline-soaked gauze pads for paddle/chest-wall interface. Current will follow the path of least resistance, so take care that cream, paste, or saline pad from one paddle

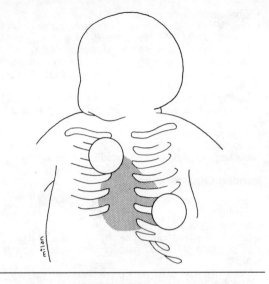

Figure C.1.

does not touch that of the other. Do NOT use
alcohol pads; serious burns can result.
- Select energy dose (joules/W-sec).
- Place one paddle to the right of the sternum just
  below the clavicle and the other paddle at the apex
  of the heart just below and lateral to the left nipple
  (Fig. C.1), **or** place one paddle anteriorly over the
  apex of the heart and the other paddle posteriorly
  below the left scapula (paddles should be in line).

- Charge defibrillator unit.
- Use APPROPRIATE mode (synchronized **or** defibrillation). REMEMBER, the defibrillator mode is used for conversion of ventricular fibrillation ONLY.
- During discharge, hold paddles firmly in position. Keep paddles flat on skin throughout procedure. Do NOT leave paddles lying on bed.
- During discharge to infant, all personnel should stand clear and avoid contact with the infant and bed.
- If not going to deliver dose, discharge unit by turning off the power, or use the disarm button while holding the paddles with metal surfaces together.

Nursing Considerations

- Obtain baseline ECG rhythm strip (12 leads if possible).
- Monitor ECG.
- Monitor oxygenation (O_2 saturation, TcO_2, and/or pO_2), blood pH, blood glucose, and infant's temperature.
- Obtain 12-lead ECG after procedure.
- Cleanse infant's skin of cream, paste, or saline.
- Document noted injury to skin (alterations in color or integrity).

NOTE Consult your particular defibrillator manual for information regarding safe and proper use.

Appendix D

Drug Information for Parents

Discharge from the neonatal intensive care unit does not mean that recovery is complete. Many infants require continued drug therapy for chronic conditions and long-term problems (e.g., apnea of prematurity, bronchopulmonary dysplasia, congenital heart disease). Teaching parents to administer necessary drugs knowledgeably and safely to their infant is an IMPORTANT part of discharge planning. A teaching plan should be devised and carried out OVER TIME to allow for assimilation of information and invaluable time to practice measuring and administering the drug/s to their infant under supervision.

Teaching Plan

- Assess parents' understanding of infant's disease state necessitating continued drug therapy.
- Develop and document individual teaching plan in infant's permanent record.
- Explain what the drug does, how it benefits their infant, and possible signs of drug toxicity or ineffectiveness.
- Teach parents how to accurately measure the drug dose using a syringe or calibrated dropper. Provide positive reinforcement and guidance.
- Teach parents how to administer the drug to THEIR infant by syringe, calibrated dropper, or nipple. BE

CONSISTENT. Provide positive reinforcement and guidance.

- Instruct the parents "when to call the doctor" and which doctor to call (cardiac vs pulmonary vs primary care physician).
- Stress the importance of follow-up with their infant's primary care doctor and specialty doctors/clinics (e.g., apnea, pulmonary, cardiac) to monitor their infant's response to the drug.
- Stress the importance of obtaining prescription refills to avoid interrupting drug therapy.
- Provide printed instructions for giving "special" drugs (e.g., digoxin, diuretics, theophylline, phenobarbital). Provide printed information in parents' primary language (e.g., Spanish). The information should include:
    - drug dose (in ml/cc, NOT mg, mcg, etc.).
    - drug schedule.
    - drug action.
    - drug storage.
    - drug administration.
    - if a dose is missed . . .
    - if a dose is vomited . . .
    - when to call the doctor.

Nursing Considerations Just Prior to Discharge

- Assure serum concentrations of drugs such as digoxin, theophylline, and phenobarbital are in the therapeutic range prior to discharge.
- Have infant on a "reasonable" schedule for drug administration allowing for uninterrupted sleep at night for infant **and** parents:

    q 12 hours: 8 AM, 8 PM.

q 8 hours: 8 AM, 4 PM, 12 midnight.
q 6 hours: 6 AM, 12 noon, 6 PM, 12 midnight.

- Provide parents with printed information for drugs such as digoxin, diuretics, theophylline, and pheno-barbital.
- Provide parents with a printed schedule of drug doses and administration times if infant is discharged on multiple drugs.
- Inform parents when last drug dose was given.

Instructions for Giving Aldactazide to Infants

NAME _____ DOCTOR _____ PHONE _____

DOSE _____ TIMES _____

What Aldactazide Does

Decreases fluid in the lungs and body by increasing your infant's urine production.

Storage of Aldactazide

- Refrigerate.
- KEEP OUT OF THE REACH OF CHILDREN.

Administration of Aldactazide

- Give EXACTLY as ordered, NEVER MORE, NEVER LESS.
- Do NOT stop the medicine unless instructed by the doctor.

- Shake bottle well before drawing up dose in the syringe.
- Use syringe to measure amount of medicine, squirt out bubbles.
- Give the medicine by mouth, by syringe or nipple.
- Give on an empty stomach or give with a small amount of formula or breast milk. Do NOT mix the medicine with the entire feeding.
- The medicine usually works within 4–6 hours, and at that time your infant should have a wetter diaper than usual.

If You Accidentally Miss a Dose

- Give the medicine as soon as you remember, up to 2 hours late.
- If more than 2 hours have passed, wait until the next scheduled time and give the regular dose. Do NOT increase the dose to make up for the missed dose.

If Your Infant Vomits the Aldactazide

- Do NOT repeat the dose if your infant vomits. Wait until the next scheduled time and give the regular dose. Do NOT increase the dose to make up for the vomited dose.

Call the Doctor If

- Your infant has vomiting and/or diarrhea for more than 24 hours (can cause dehydration and may require a temporary adjustment of the medicine).
- Your infant shows signs of dehydration, which include sunken fontanelle (the soft spot on top of infant's head), dryness inside of mouth, fast heart

rate (greater than 180 beats per minute), fewer wet diapers, and dark-colored urine.
- Your infant shows signs of fluid in the lungs and body, which include increased breathing rate (greater than 60 breaths per minute) or labored breathing (pulling in of chest with breaths), increased irritability or restlessness, puffiness (especially around the eyes), and blue color (usually first seen about the lips, mouth, and eyes).

Instructions for Giving Digoxin (Lanoxin) to Infants

NAME _____ DOCTOR _____ PHONE _____

DOSE _____ TIMES _____

What Digoxin Does

Slows down your infant's heart and makes it pump blood more efficiently.

Storage of Digoxin

- Store at room temperature.
- KEEP OUT OF THE REACH OF CHILDREN, preferably in a locked cabinet.

Administration of Digoxin

- Give EXACTLY as ordered, NEVER MORE, NEVER LESS.
- Give regularly, do NOT vary time by more than 1 or 2 hours if possible.

- Do NOT stop the medicine unless instructed by the doctor.
- Use premeasured dropper or syringe to measure amount of medicine, squirt out bubbles.
- Give the medicine by mouth, by dropper or syringe, on an empty stomach.
- Do NOT mix with formula, breast milk, or foods.

If You Accidentally Miss a Dose

- Give the medicine as soon as you remember, up to 6 hours late.
- If more than 6 hours have passed, wait until the next scheduled time and give the regular dose. Do NOT increase the dose to make up for the missed dose.
- If you miss more than two doses in a row, call the cardiology (heart) doctor.

If Your Infant Vomits the Digoxin

- Do NOT repeat the dose if vomiting occurs AFTER 5 minutes from the time the digoxin was given.
- Repeat the dose ONLY ONE TIME if vomiting occurs WITHIN 5 minutes from the time the digoxin was given. If you are not sure, do NOT give the dose.
- If two doses are missed because of vomiting, call the cardiology (heart) doctor.

Call the Cardiology (Heart) Doctor if Infant Shows Signs of Heart Failure

- Increased irritability or restlessness.
- Increased breathing rate (greater than 60 breaths

per minute) or labored breathing (pulling in of chest
with breaths).
- Increased sweating.
- Puffiness, especially around the eyes.
- Poor suck and feeding. Fatigue with feeding.
- Cyanosis (blue color), usually first seen about lips,
  mouth, and eyes.

Instructions for Giving Furosemide (Lasix) to Infants

NAME _____ DOCTOR _____ PHONE _____

DOSE _____ TIMES _____

What Lasix Does

Decreases fluid in the lungs and body by increasing
your infant's urine production.

Storage of Lasix

- Store at room temperature.
- KEEP OUT OF THE REACH OF CHILDREN.

Administration of Lasix

- Give EXACTLY as ordered, NEVER MORE, NEVER
  LESS.
- Do NOT stop the medicine unless instructed by the
  doctor.
- Use premeasured dropper or syringe to measure
  amount of medicine, squirt out bubbles.
- Give the medicine by mouth, by dropper, syringe,
  or nipple.

- Give on an empty stomach or give with a small amount of formula or breast milk. Do NOT mix the medicine with the entire feeding.
- The medicine usually works within 1–2 hours, and at that time your infant should have a wetter diaper than usual.

If You Accidentally Miss a Dose

- If your infant takes one dose a day, give the medicine as soon as you remember, up to 12 hours late. If more than 12 hours have passed, wait until the next scheduled time and give the regular dose.
- If your infant takes more than one dose a day, give the medicine as soon as you remember, up to 2 hours late. If more than 2 hours have passed, wait until the next scheduled time and give the regular dose.
- Do NOT increase the dose to make up for the missed dose.

If Your Infant Vomits the Lasix

- Do NOT repeat the dose if your infant vomits. Wait until the next scheduled time and give the regular dose. Do NOT increase the dose to make up for the vomited dose.

Call the Doctor If

- Your infant has vomiting and/or diarrhea for more than 24 hours (can cause dehydration and may require a temporary adjustment of the medicine).
- Your infant shows signs of dehydration, which include sunken fontanelle (the soft spot on top of infant's head), dryness inside of mouth, fast heart

rate (greater than 180 beats per minute), fewer wet diapers, and dark-colored urine.
- Your infant shows signs of fluid in the lungs and body, which include increased breathing rate (greater than 60 breaths per minute) or labored breathing (pulling in of chest with breaths), increased irritability or restlessness, puffiness (especially around the eyes), and blue color (usually first seen about the lips, mouth, and eyes).

Instructions for Giving Phenobarbital to Infants

NAME _____ DOCTOR _____ PHONE _____

DOSE _____ TIMES _____

What Phenobarbital Does

Controls your infant's seizures.

Storage of Phenobarbital

- Store at room temperature.
- Keep bottle tightly closed.
- KEEP OUT OF THE REACH OF CHILDREN.

Administration of Phenobarbital

- Give EXACTLY as ordered, NEVER MORE, NEVER LESS.
- Do NOT stop the medicine unless instructed by the doctor.
- Use syringe to measure the amount of medicine, squirt out bubbles.

- Give the medicine slowly by mouth, with the syringe or nipple.
- Give the medicine with at least an equal amount of formula or breast milk. Do NOT mix the medicine with the entire feeding. Do NOT give on an empty stomach.

If You Accidentally Miss a Dose

- Give the medicine as soon as you remember, up to 6 hours late.
- If more than 6 hours have passed, wait until the next scheduled time and give the regular dose. Do NOT increase the dose to make up for the missed dose.

If Your Infant Vomits the Phenobarbital

- Do NOT repeat the dose if vomiting occurs AFTER 15 minutes from the time the phenobarbital was given.
- Repeat the dose ONLY ONE TIME if vomiting occurs WITHIN 15 minutes from the time the phenobarbital was given.
- If two doses are missed because of vomiting, call the doctor.

Call the Doctor If

- Your infant is floppy, unusually sleepy, or difficult to arouse.
- Your infant has a poor suck or appetite.
- Your infant has shallow breathing.
- You observe seizure activity (e.g., unusual eye or mouth movements, rhythmic or jerky movements of

arms and/or legs, and abnormal posturing of body, arms, and/or legs).

Instructions for Giving Theophylline to Infants

NAME _____ DOCTOR _____ PHONE _____

DOSE _____ TIMES _____

What Theophylline Does

Stimulates your infant's breathing and keeps the airways in the lungs open.

Storage of Theophylline

- Store at room temperature.
- KEEP OUT OF THE REACH OF CHILDREN.

Administration of Theophylline

- Give EXACTLY as ordered, NEVER MORE, NEVER LESS.
- Do NOT stop the medicine unless instructed by the doctor.
- Use syringe to measure the amount of medicine, squirt out bubbles.
- Give the medicine by mouth, with the syringe or nipple.
- Give the medicine with a small amount of formula or breast milk. Do NOT mix the medicine with the entire feeding.

If You Accidentally Miss a Dose

- Give the medicine as soon as you remember, up to 2 hours late.
- If more than 2 hours have passed, wait until the next scheduled time and give the regular dose. Do NOT increase the dose to make up for the missed dose.

If Your Infant Vomits the Theophylline

- Do NOT repeat the dose if your infant vomits. Wait until the next scheduled time and give the regular dose. Do NOT increase the dose to make up for the vomited dose.
- If three doses are missed because of vomiting, call the doctor. Vomiting may be a sign of toxicity.

Call the Doctor If

- Your infant's heart rate is greater than 180 beats per minute when your infant is ASLEEP. Check your infant's heart rate once a day while he/she is asleep. Gently feel the pulse on the inside of your infant's arm (as you were shown in your CPR class).
- Your infant is unusually irritable.
- Your infant has missed three doses of medicine because of vomiting.
- Your baby has apnea and bradycardia requiring your intervention.

Appendix E

Drugs in Breast Milk

The presence of drugs in human breast milk is a subject of concern to health care practitioners and to parents considering breast-feeding their infant. Breast-feeding is currently enjoying a wave of popularity. Research on the subject must answer three basic questions. First, what factors affect the passage of a drug into breast milk? Second, does the drug appear in breast milk? Third, is its presence of clinical significance to the infant?

Drug passage into breast milk is affected by the drug's molecular weight, lipid solubility, pH and degree of ionization, and protein binding capacity.

Molecular Weight

Small (molecular weight <200 units), nonionic substances may enter breast milk by simple diffusion through pores in mammary epithelial cell walls. Larger molecules must be transported across cell membranes to enter the mammary gland. Most drugs have a molecular weight <200 units and diffuse through the pores.

Lipid Solubility

Drugs must have solubility in both water and lipid to penetrate the mammary gland and remain in breast milk. Lipid-soluble drugs may concentrate in milk with its high fat content. The fat content of milk varies throughout the day, and varies according to how long an infant has been breast-feeding.

pH and Degree of Ionization

Most drugs are weak acids or weak bases, and as such, will ionize at a given pH. The pKa is the pH at which a weak acid or base is 50% ionized. Only non-ionized drugs will cross cell membranes. The typical pH of blood is ~7.4. The typical pH of human breast milk is ~7.0. This favors weak bases concentrating in breast milk. Weak bases that are nonionized at a pH of 7.4 in the blood pass into breast milk and may ionize in the relatively acidic (pH 7.0) environment of breast milk. These ionized drugs cannot cross cell membranes and tend to remain in breast milk. This is referred to as "ion trapping." Conversely, weak acids that are ionized at a pH of 7.4 in the blood cannot pass into breast milk as easily.

Protein Binding

Protein binding affects drug passage into breast milk. A drug that is highly protein bound in the serum will only have a small free (unbound) fraction available to cross cell membranes and enter breast milk.

Finally, some endogenous substances are actively transported into breast milk. Examples of these are amino acids, glucose, and calcium. No known drugs are actively transported in humans.

Typically, drug concentrations in breast milk are not constant, rising and falling in much the same way that serum drug concentrations rise and fall. The ratio of drug concentration in the milk to the simultaneous drug concentration in the maternal plasma is called the "milk-plasma ratio." The milk-plasma ratio is of little practical value in deciding if a mother should breast-feed or not. The serum concentration curve is not parallel with the breast milk concentration curve, and reported ratios will vary depending upon when the drug concentrations were drawn.

Certain drugs, when taken by the mother, are an absolute contraindication to breast-feeding. For most drugs, however, the drug dose that the infant receives while breast-feeding, and its potential effect, will determine whether breast-feeding is advisable. Any ingested substance must be absorbed from the infant's GI tract to produce a pharmacologic effect. Nursing should be avoided when drug concentrations in breast milk are highest. A nursing mother's drug therapy should be temporarily interrupted if possible, or discontinued if drug therapy is not absolutely necessary. Frequently, an alternative drug from the same drug class may be equally effective in the mother but appear in her breast milk in low enough concentrations to allow breast-feeding.

Newborn infants, especially preterm infants, have immature liver and renal clearance mechanisms, predisposing them to accumulate drugs. A summary of various drugs and their possible impact on breast-feeding infants is presented in Table E.1.

Table E.1.
Drugs and Breast-feeding

Drug or Drug Class	Breast-feeding Recommended	Possible Effect on Infant	Comments
Acetaminophen	Yes	No effect.	Take after nursing.
Acyclovir	No	Bone marrow suppression.	High levels in milk.
Alcohol	±	CNS depression when large amounts consumed.	Do not nurse for several hours after consumption (1 hour/drink).
Amantadine	No	Vomiting. Urinary retention. Skin rash.	CONTRAINDICATED by manufacturer.
Aminoglycosides (amikacin, gentamicin, tobramycin)	Yes	Change in GI flora. Diarrhea. Thrush.	Present in breast milk but not absorbed from infant's GI tract.
Aminophylline	Yes	Wakefulness. Irritability.	Sustained-release forms or continuous IV drip will increase dose to infant.

Drug	Safe	Effects	Comments
Amphetamines	No	Wakefulness. Irritability.	Present in breast milk, amount may vary.
Antidepressants (amitriptyline, doxepin, imipramine, trazodone)	±	Respiratory depression.	Poorly studied. Low concentration in breast milk. Long-term effects unknown. Avoid doxepin, trazodone, and newer drugs.
Antihistamines	Yes	Drowsiness.	May decrease milk flow. Avoid sustained-release forms.
Aspirin	±	No effect with low dose.	High doses (650 mg q 4 hours) may cause metabolic acidosis.
Barbiturates	Yes	Drowsiness. May induce liver enzymes.	Present in breast milk, probably not enough to cause CNS effects.
Benzodiazepines	No	Drowsiness. CNS depression.	May accumulate in infants due to immature liver enzymes. Diazepam is worst in class.
β-Blockers (atenolol, labe-	Yes	Bradycardia. Hypotension.	Low levels in milk with propranolol, meto-

Table E.1.
Drugs and Breast-feeding—continued

Drug or Drug Class	Breast-feeding Recommended	Possible Effect on Infant	Comments
talol, metoprolol, propranolol)			prolol, and labetalol. High levels with atenolol, nadolol.
Caffeine	Yes	Jitteriness with high intake.	Small amounts in milk.
Captopril	Yes	No apparent effect.	Small amounts in milk.
Carbamazepine	Yes	No apparent effect.	Small amounts in milk.
Cephalosporins	Yes	Change in GI flora. Diarrhea.	Sensitivity? Observe for rash, thrush, diarrhea.
Chloral hydrate	Yes	Sedation. Drowsiness.	≥50% of maternal serum concentration found in milk.
Chloramphenicol	No	Bone marrow suppression.	CONTRAINDICATED.
Cimetidine	No	Unknown.	pKa causes concentration in breast milk.

Drug		Effect	Notes
Cocaine	No	CNS excitement. Agitation.	CONTRAINDICATED.
Corticosteroids (dexamethasone, hydrocortisone, prednisolone, prednisone)	Yes	HPA-axis suppression not likely.	Prednisolone best in this class.
Chemotherapy/ Antineoplastics	No	Bone marrow suppression.	CONTRAINDICATED.
Digoxin	Yes	No effect.	Insignificant amounts in milk.
Ergot alkaloids	No	Ergotism in infants. GI irritation.	CONTRAINDICATED. Take after nursing.
Erythromycin	Yes		
Estrogens	See Oral Contraceptives		
Furosemide	Yes	No effect.	Not found in milk. Can suppress lactation with high doses.
Haloperidol	No	Long-term effect unknown.	Small amounts in milk.
Heparin	Yes	No effect.	Heparin molecule is

Table E.1.
Drugs and Breast-feeding—continued

Drug or Drug Class	Breast-feeding Recommended	Possible Effect on Infant	Comments
			too large to pass into milk.
Hydralazine	Yes	No effect with short-term use. Long-term?	Monitor infant for tachycardia and hypotension.
Insulin	Yes	No effect.	Insulin in milk not absorbed from infant's GI tract.
Isoniazid	Yes	Toxic to liver? (allergic reaction)	Concentration in milk equal to maternal serum concentrations.
Lithium	No	Vomiting. Polyuria.	CONTRAINDICATED.
LSD	No	CNS toxicity.	CONTRAINDICATED.
Marijuana	No	CNS effects.	CONTRAINDICATED.
Methimazole	No	Thyroid suppression.	CONTRAINDICATED.
Metronidazole	No	Poor feeding. Vomiting	CONTRAINDICATED for 24–48 hours after last dose.

Drug	Safe?	Effects	Comments
Nonsteroidal anti-inflammatory agents	Yes	GI irritation. Vomiting.	Ibuprofen has lowest milk levels in this class. Avoid longer-acting agents.
Opiates (heroin, methadone, codeine, meperidine, morphine, oxycodone, propoxyphene)	Yes	CNS depression. Drowsiness.	Codeine, meperidine, morphine, oxycodone, or propoxyphene: nurse prior to dose. Methadone: do not nurse for 4–6 hours after dose. Heroin: CONTRAINDICATED.
Oral contraceptives Estrogens and combinations	No	Gynecomastia. Jaundice.	Avoid breast-feeding or choose alternative methods of birth control. Estrogens decrease lactation.
Progestins alone	Yes		
Penicillins (ampicillin, dicloxacillin,	Yes	Sensitization?	Weigh breast-feeding vs risk of sensitization. Observe for thrush or

Table E.1.
Drugs and Breast-feeding—continued

Drug or Drug Class	Breast-feeding Recommended	Possible Effect on Infant	Comments
methicillin, nafcillin, penicillin, etc.)			diarrhea.
Phenytoin	Yes	May induce liver enzymes. Rash. Liver toxicity.	Small amounts in milk, insufficient for toxic levels.
Primidone	Yes	Drowsiness.	Metabolite (phenobarbital) may reach significant levels in milk.
Propylthiouracil	Yes	Thyroid suppression unlikely.	Monitor infant's thyroid function if breast-feeding.
Quinidine	Yes	No effect.	Low concentration in milk.
Radiopharmaceuticals	No	Possible bone marrow suppression.	CONTRAINDICATED.
Rifampin	Yes	No effect.	Not found in milk.

Memory Bank for Neonatal Drugs

Drug	Excreted in milk	Effect on infant	Comment
Spironolactone	Yes	No apparent effect.	Low concentration in milk.
Sulfonamides	±	Hemolysis in G6PD-deficient infants. Increased susceptibility to kernicterus in infants <2 month and preterm infants.	Contraindicated in G6PD deficiency. Use sulfisoxazole or sulfamethoxazole if maternal treatment with sulfonamides is needed.
Tetracyclines	±	Mottling of teeth?	Avoid breast-feeding or choose alternative drug.
Theophylline	See Aminophylline		
Thiazides	Yes	Diuresis. Electrolyte imbalance unlikely.	Low doses may not affect infant.
Thyroid drugs	Yes	Hyperthyroid effects.	Replacement doses probably will not affect infant.
Tranquilizers (chlorpromazine, fluphenazine, haloperi-	Yes	Drowsiness. Extrapyramidal signs?	Low levels in milk.

Appendix E: Drugs in Breast Milk

Table E.1.
Drugs and Breast-feeding—continued

Drug or Drug Class	Breast-feeding Recommended	Possible Effect on Infant	Comments
dol, perphena-zine, thi-oridazine)			
Warfarin	Yes	No effect.	Levels in milk not sig-nificant with maternal doses 10 mg/day or less.

NOTE
This table was compiled from review of several widely used references on drugs in human breast milk. If conflicting data were reported, authors' recommendations have taken a conservative view of the available data.

Laboratory Values

Normal values may vary with gestational and postnatal age of infant, and may vary slightly with different laboratories.

Chemistry Values

Albumin	Preterm	2.5–4.5 gm/dl	
	Term	2.5–5.0 gm/dl	
	Infant	4–5 gm/dl	
Ammonia	Newborn	90–150 µg/dl	
	1 month	29–70 µg/dl	
Bicarbonate	Preterm	18–26 mEq/L	
	Term	20–26 mEq/L	
Bilirubin, total		Preterm	Term
	Cord	< 2.8 mg/dl	< 2.8 mg/dl
	24 hours	1–6 mg/dl	2–6 mg/dl
	48 hours	6–8 mg/dl	6–7 mg/dl
	3–5 days	10–12 mg/dl	4–6 mg/dl
	≥ 1 month	< 1.5 mg/dl	≤ 1.5 mg/dl
Bilirubin, direct	< 0.5 mg/dl		
Calcium, total	Preterm	6–10 mg/dl	
	Term	7–12 mg/dl	
	Infant	8.5–11 mg/dl	
Calcium, ionized	2.5–5 mg/dl		

Chloride	Preterm	95–110 mEq/L
	Term	96–107 mEq/L
	Infant	98–106 mEq/L
Creatinine (serum)	Newborn	0.2–1.4 mg/dl
	Infant	≤ 0.6 mg/dl
Cholesterol	Newborn	50–120 mg/dl
	Infant	65–175 mg/dl
Glucose	Preterm	20–65 mg/dl
	Term	30–60 mg/dl
	Infant	60–100 mg/dl
Immunoglobulin G (IgG)	Newborn	900–1500 mg/dl
	1–3 months	250–550 mg/dl
	4–6 months	300–600 mg/dl
Magnesium		1.5–2.8 mEq/L
Osmolality (serum)		285–295 mOsm/L
Phosphatase, alkaline	Infant	150–400 units/L
Phosphorous	Preterm	5.5–8 mg/dl
	Term	5–8 mg/dl
	Infant	5–9.5 mg/dl
Potassium	Newborn	3.5–6 mEq/L
	Infant	3.5–5 mEq/L
Protein, total	Preterm	4–5 gm/dl
	Term	5–7 gm/dl
	Infant	4–7 gm/dl
Sodium	Newborn	135–145 mEq/L
	Infant	140–145 mEq/L
SGOT		24–81 units/L

SGPT   0–54 units/L

Triglyceride   30–100 mg/dl

**Urea nitrogen
(blood)**   5–25 mg/dl

Hematology Values

Blood   Newborn   80–85 ml/kg
volume   > 1 month 75 ml/kg

**Absolute neutrophil
count (ANC)**
              Newborn   3500–6000/mm³

Fibrinogen   150–400 mg/dl

Hematocrit		Preterm	Term
	Birth	> 45%	50–65%
	6–8 weeks	25–28%	35%

Hemoglobin		Preterm	Term
	Birth	14–15 gm/dl	17–19 gm/dl
	6–8 weeks	8–10 gm/dl	11–12 gm/dl

Leukocytes, total	Newborn	1 Week	1 Month
× 1000/mm³	9–30	5–21	5–19.5
Neutrophils, total	60–70%	45%	35%
segmented	47% ± 15	34%	25% ± 10
bands	14% ± 4	11%	9% ± 3
Lymphocytes	30–40%	41%	56%
Monocytes	6%	9%	7%
Eosinophils	2%	4%	3%

Appendix F: Laboratory Values   **301**

Nucleated RBCs		Preterm	Term
	Birth	1000–5000/ mm³	up to 500/ mm³
	≥ 1 week	0	0

Partial thrombo- plastin time (PTT)

	Preterm	2 × control
	Term	< 10 seconds > control

Platelet count 100,000–300,000/mm³

Prothrombin time (PT)	Preterm	10 seconds > control
	Term	2–3 seconds > control

Reticulocyte count		Preterm	Term
	< 1 week	5–10%	3–7%
	> 1 week	1–4%	0.5–1%
	2 months	3–6%	1.8%

Lung Profile, Normal Pregnancy

	Immature	Premature	Intermediate	Mature with Caution	Mature
L/S	< 1	1.0–1.5	1.5–1.9	2.0–2.2	2.5–3.8
% ptt	10–40	< 40	40–50	> 50	
% PI	trace–5	5–12	12–20	20–25	20–15
% PG	0	0	0	0–2	2–10
Weeks	26–30	30–34	34–35	35–36	37–40

L/S   lecithin/sphingomyelin ratio
ptt   disaturated phosphatidylcholine
PI   phosphatidylinositol
PG   phosphatidylglycerol

Weights and Measures

Metric Weight Equivalents

1 kilogram (kg) = 1000 grams
1 gram (gm) = 1000 milligrams
1 milligram (mg) = 0.001 gram
1 microgram (mcg, μg) = 0.001 milligram
1 nanogram (ng) = 0.001 microgram

Metric Volume Equivalents

1 liter (L) = 1000 milliliters (ml)
1 deciliter (dl) = 100 milliliters

Weight/Volume Equivalents

1 mg/dl = 10 mcg/ml
1 mg/dl = 1 mg%

Conversion Equivalents

1 ounce (oz) = 28.35 grams
1 pound (lb) = 453.6 grams
1 kilogram (kg) = 2.2 pounds

Temperature Equivalents

CENTI-GRADE	FAHREN-HEIT	CENTI-GRADE	FAHREN-HEIT
35.0	95.0	37.6	99.6
35.2	95.4	37.8	100.0
35.4	95.7	38.0	100.4
35.6	96.1	38.2	100.7
35.8	96.4	38.4	101.1
36.0	96.8	38.6	101.4
36.2	97.1	38.8	101.8
36.4	97.5	39.0	102.2
36.6	97.8	39.2	102.5
36.8	98.2	39.4	102.9
37.0	98.6	39.6	103.2
37.2	98.9	39.8	103.6
37.4	99.3	40.0	104.0

Centigrade to Fahrenheit

$[(°C \times 9) \div 5] + 32 = °F$

Fahrenheit to Centigrade

$5 \times (°F - 32) \div 9 = °C$

Conversion of Pounds and Ounces to Grams

	Pounds (lb)										
Ounces (oz)	0	1	2	3	4	5	6	7	8	9	10
0	0	454	907	1361	1814	2268	2722	3175	3629	4082	4536
1	28	482	936	1389	1843	2296	2750	3203	3657	4111	4564
2	57	510	964	1417	1871	2325	2778	3232	3685	4139	4593
3	85	539	992	1446	1899	2353	2807	3260	3714	4167	4621
4	113	567	1021	1474	1928	2381	2835	3289	3742	4196	4649
5	142	595	1049	1503	1956	2410	2863	3317	3770	4224	4678
6	170	624	1077	1531	1984	2438	2892	3345	3799	4252	4706
7	198	652	1106	1559	2013	2466	2920	3374	3827	4281	4734
8	227	680	1134	1588	2041	2495	2948	3402	3856	4309	4763
9	255	709	1162	1616	2070	2523	2977	3430	3884	4337	4791
10	283	737	1191	1644	2098	2551	3005	3459	3912	4366	4819
11	312	765	1219	1673	2126	2580	3033	3487	3941	4394	4848
12	340	794	1247	1701	2155	2608	3062	3515	3969	4423	4876
13	369	822	1276	1729	2183	2637	3090	3544	3997	4451	4904
14	397	850	1304	1758	2211	2665	3118	3752	4026	4479	4933
15	425	879	1332	1786	2240	2693	3147	3600	4054	4508	4961

Abbreviations

AAP	American Academy of Pediatrics
ACT	activated clotting time
ASAP	as soon as possible
BP	blood pressure
BPD	bronchopulmonary dysplasia
bpm	beats per minute
BUN	blood urea nitrogen
Ca^{2+}	elemental calcium
CBC	complete blood count
CHF	congestive heart failure
CNS	central nervous system
CV	cardiovascular
CVP	central venous pressure
DA	ductus arteriosus
D5W	dextrose 5% in water
ECG	electrocardiogram
EKG	electrocardiogram
ET	endotracheal
ETT	endotracheal tube
FP	freezing point
GE	gastroesophageal
GI	gastrointestinal
HBsAg	hepatitis B surface antigen
HR	heart rate
IC	intracardiac
Ig	immunoglobulin
IM	intramuscular(ly)

IU	international unit(s)
IV	intravenous(ly)
IVH	intraventricular hemorrhage
IVIG	intravenous immune globulin
LDH	lactic dehydrogenase
NaCl	sodium chloride
NS	normal saline
0.45% NaCl	half normal saline
0.9% NaCl	normal saline
PDA	patent ductus arteriosus
PO	by mouth
PR	by recturn
prn	as needed
PT	prothrombin time
PTT	partial thromboplastin time
q	each
qd	every day
RDA	recommended daily allowance
RDS	respiratory distress syndrome
RR	respiratory rate
SGOT	serum glutamic oxaloacetic transaminase
SGPT	serum glutamic pyruvic transaminase
SQ	subcutaneous(ly)
$TcCO_2$	transcutaneous CO_2
TcO_2	transcutaneous O_2
TPN	total parenteral nutrition
UAC	umbilical arterial catheter
UVC	umbilical venous catheter
VLBW	very low birth weight
W-sec	watt-second

Bibliography

Adams FH, Emmanouilides GC (eds): *Moss' Heart Disease in Infants, Children, and Adolescents,* ed 4. Baltimore, Williams & Wilkins, 1989.

American Academy of Pediatrics, Committee on Drugs: Emergency drug doses for infants and children. *Pediatrics* 81: 462–465, 1988.

American Academy of Pediatrics, Committee on Infectious Diseases: *Report of the Committee on Infectious Diseases,* ed 21. Evanston, IL, American Academy of Pediatrics, 1988.

American Academy of Pediatrics, Committee on Nutrition: Nutritional needs of preterm infants. In Forbes GB (ed): *Pediatric Nutrition Handbook,* ed 2. Evanston, IL, American Academy of Pediatrics, 1985, p 66.

Aranda JV, Turmen T: Methylxanthines in apnea of prematurity. *Clin Perinatol* 6: 87–108, 1979.

Artman M, Graham TP: Congestive heart failure in infancy: Recognition and management. *Am Heart J* 103: 1040–1054, 1982.

Artman M, Graham TP: Guidelines for vasodilator therapy of congestive heart failure in infants and children. *Am Heart J* 113: 994–1005, 1987.

Atkinson HC, Begg EJ, Darlow BA: Drugs in human milk, clinical pharmacokinetic considerations. *Clin Pharmacokinet* 14: 217–240, 1988.

Avery GB (ed): *Neonatology: Pathophysiology and Management of the Newborn,* ed 3. Philadelphia, JB Lippincott Co, 1987.

Avery GB, Fletcher AB, Kaplan M, Brundo DS: Controlled trial of dexamethasone in respirator-dependent infants with bronchopulmonary dysplasia. *Pediatrics* 75: 106–111, 1985.

Bankier A, Turner M, Hopkins IJ: Pyridoxine dependent seizures—a wider clinical spectrum. *Arch Dis Child* 58: 415–418, 1983.

Barrington KJ, Finer NN, Peters KL, Barton J: Physiologic effects of doxapram in idiopathic apnea of prematurity. *J Pediatr* 108: 124–129, 1986.

Benitez WE, Frankel LR, Stevenson DK: The pharmacology of neonatal resuscitation and cardiopulmonary intensive care. Part 1—Immediate resuscitation. *West J Med* 144: 704–709, 1986.

Benitez WE, Frankel LR, Stevenson DK: The pharmacology of neonatal resuscitation and cardiopulmonary intensive care. Part II—Extended intensive care. *West J Med* 145: 47–51, 1986.

Benitez WE, Malachowski N, Cohen RS, Stevenson DK, Ariagno RL, Sunshine P: Use of sodium nitroprusside in neonates: efficacy and safety. *J Pediatr* 106: 102–110, 1985.

Blanchard PW, Brown TM, Coates AL: Pharmacotherapy in bronchopulmonary dysplasia. *Clin Perinatol* 14: 881–910, 1987.

Blumer JL, Rothstein FC, Kaplan BS, Yamashita TS, Eshelman FN, Myers CM, Reed MD: Pharmacokinetic determination of ranitidine pharmacodynamics in pediatric ulcer disease. *J Pediatr* 107: 301–306, 1985.

Brixen-Rasmussen L, Halgrener J, Jorgensen A: Amitriptyline and nortriptyline excretion in human breast milk. *Psychopharmacology* 76: 94–95, 1982.

Brown WI, Buist NRM, Gipson HT, et al: Fatal benzyl alcohol poisoning in a neonatal intensive care unit. *Lancet* 1: 1250–1251, 1982.

Candian Society of Hospital Pharmacists: *Extemporaneous Oral Liquid Dosage Preparations.* Toronto, Candian Society of Hospital Pharmacists, 1988.

Bibliography

Cloherty JP, Stark AR (eds): *Manual of Neonatal Care,* ed 2. Boston, Little, Brown & Co, 1985.

Costarino AT, Polin RA: Neuromuscular relaxants in the neonate. *Clin Perinatol* 14: 965–989, 1987.

Crelin ES: *Anatomy of the Newborn: An Atlas.* Philadelphia, Lea & Febiger, 1969.

Chirico G, Rondini G, Plebani A, et al: Intravenous gammaglobulin therapy for prophylaxis of infection in high risk neonates. *J Pediatr* 110: 437–442, 1987.

Deshmukh A, Wittert W, Schnizler E, Mangurten HH: Lorazepam in the treatment of refractory neonatal seizures, a pilot study. *Am J Dis Child* 140: 1042–1044, 1986.

Dombrowski SR (ed): *Extemporaneous Formulations.* Bethesda, MD, American Society of Hospital Pharmacists, 1987.

Driscoll DJ: Use of inotropic and chronotropic agents in the newborn. *Clin Perinatol* 14: 931–949, 1987.

Drug manufacturer's medication package inserts.

Ernst JA, Williams JM, Glick MR, Lemons JA: Osmolality of substances used in the intensive care nursery. *Pediatrics* 72: 347–352, 1983.

Fanaroff AA, Martin RJ (eds): *Neonatal-Perinatal Medicine, Diseases of the Fetus and Infant,* ed 4. St. Louis, CV Mosby Co, 1987.

Finnegan LP: Neonatal abstinence. In Nelson N (ed): *Current Therapy in Neonatal-Perinatal Medicine 1985–1986.* Toronto, BC Decker Inc, 1985, p 262.

Fuller R: Cardiac function and the neonatal EKG, Part I: Introduction to neonatal EKGs. *Neonatal Netw* 7: 47–51, 1989.

Gershanik JJ, Boecler G, George W, et al: The gasping syndrome: Benzyl alcohol (BA) poisoning? *Clin Res* 29: 895, 1981.

Grasela TH Jr, Donn SM: Neonatal population pharmacokinetics of phenobarbital derived from routine clinical data. *Dev Pharmacol Ther* 8: 374–383, 1985.

Green TP: The pharmacologic basis of diuretic therapy in the newborn. *Clin Perinatol* 14: 951–964, 1987.

Hargrove C: Administration of IV medications in the NICU: The development of a procedure. *Neonatal Netw* 6: 41–49, 1987.

Harper RG, Yoon JJ: *Handbook of Neonatology,* ed 2. Chicago, Year Book Medical Publishers, Inc, 1987.

Hayakawa F, Hakamada S, Kuno K, Nakashima T, Miyachi Y: Doxapram in the treatment of idiopathic apnea of prematurity: desirable dose and serum concentration. *J Pediatr* 109: 138–140, 1986.

Kearn GL, Jacobs RF, Thomas BR, Darville TL, Trang JM: Cefotaxime and desacetylcefotaxime pharmacokinetics in very low birth weight neonates. *J Pediatr* 114: 461–467, 1989.

Klaus MH, Fanaroff AA: *Care of the High-Risk Neonate,* ed 3. Philadelphia, WB Saunders Co, 1986.

Knoben JE, Anderson PO (eds): *Handbook of Clinical Drug Data,* ed 6. Hamilton, IL, Drug Intelligence Publications Inc, 1988.

Koren G, Lau A, Klein J, Golas C, Bologa-Campeanu M, Soldin S, MacLeod SM, Prober C: Pharmacokinetics and adverse effects of amphotericin B in infants and children. *J Pediatr* 113: 559–563, 1988.

Koren G, Zarfin Y, Maresky D, Spiro TE, MacLeod SM: Pharmacokinetics of intravenous clindamycin in newborn infants. *Pediatr Pharmacol* 5: 287–292, 1986.

Kulovich MV, Hallman MB, Gluck L: The long profile, I. Normal pregnancy. *Am J Obstet Gynecol* 135: 57–63, 1979.

Kumar SP: Adverse drug reactions in the newborn. *Ann Clin Lab Sci* 15: 195–203, 1985.

Low LCK, Lang J, Alexander WD: Excretion of carbimazole and propylthiouracil in breast milk (Letter). *Lancet* 2: 1011, 1979.

Marchal F, Bairam A, Vert P: Neonatal apnea and apneic syndromes. *Clin Perinatol* 14: 509–529, 1987.

Mardoum R, Bejar R, McFeely E, Peterson B, Merritt TA: Controlled study of the effects of indomethacin on the cerebral blood flow velocities in the newborn infant. *Pediatr Res* 23: 554 A, 1988.

McCracken GH, Nelson JD: *Antimicrobial Therapy for Newborns,* ed 2. New York, Grune & Stratton, 1983.

McEvoy GK (ed): *Drug Information 88.* Bethesda, MD, American Society of Hospital Pharmacists Inc, 1988.

Miller ME, Cohn RD, Burghart PH: Hydrochlorothiazide disposition in a mother and her breast-fed infant. *J Pediatr* 101: 789–791, 1982.

Mirochnick MH, Miceli JJ, Kramer PA, Chapron DJ, Raye JR: Furosemide pharmacokinetics in very low birth-weight infants. *J Pediatr* 112: 653–657, 1988.

Moller JH, Neal WA: *Heart Disease in Infancy.* New York, Appleton-Century-Crofts, 1981.

Morett LA, Ortega R: Pulmonary hypertension in the fetus, the newborn and the child. *Clin Perinatol* 14: 227–242, 1987.

Nathan DG, Oski FA: *Hematology of Infancy and Child-hood* (Vol 2), ed 3. Philadelphia, WB Saunders Co, 1987.

Nelson JD: *Pocketbook of Pediatric Antimicrobial Therapy,* ed 6. Baltimore, Williams & Wilkins, 1985.

Noerr B: Commonly used drugs in the neonatal intensive care setting. *Neonatal Netw* 2: 42–47, 1984.

Noya FJ, Rench MA, Garcia-Prats JA, Jones TM, Baker CJ: Disposition of an immunoglobulin intravenous preparation in very low birth weight neonates. *J Pediatr* 112: 278–283, 1988.

Nugent SK, Laravuso R, Rogers MC. Pharmacology and use of muscle relaxants in infants and children. *J Pediatr* 94: 481–487, 1979.

Ohio Neonatal Nutritionists: *Nutritional Care for High Risk Newborns.* Philadelphia, George F Strickley Co, 1985.

PDR (Physician's Desk Reference) ed 43. Oradell, NJ, Medical Economics Company Inc, 1989.

Peckham GJ: Patent ductus arteriosus. In Nelson NM (ed): *Current Therapy in Neonatal-Perinatal Medicine 1985–1986*. Toronto, BC Decker Inc, 1985, p 273.

Perez-Reyes M, Wall ME: Presence of Δ^9-tetrahydrocannabinol in human milk. *N Engl J Med* 307:819–820, 1982.

Pickoff AS, Gelband H: Cardiac arrhythmias and conduction disturbances. In Nelson NM (ed): *Current Therapy in Neonatal-Perinatal Medicine 1985–1986*. Toronto, BC Decker Inc, 1985, p 150.

Pickoff AS, Singh S, Gelband H: The medical management of cardiac arrhythmias. In Roberts NK, Gelband H (eds): *Cardiac Arrhythmias in the Neonate, Infant and Child*, ed 2. Norwalk, CT, Appleton-Century-Crofts, 1983, p 297.

Roberts RJ: *Drug Therapy in Infants, Pharmacologic Principles and Clinical Experience*. Philadelphia, WB Saunders Co, 1984.

Roberts RJ: Principles of neonatal pharmacology. In Avery ME, Taeusch HW (eds): *Schaffer's Diseases of the Newborn*. Philadelphia, WB Saunders Co, 1984, p 950.

Rowe PC (ed): *The Harriet Lane Handbook*, ed 11. Chicago, Year Book Medical Publishers, Inc, 1987.

Schechter NL: Pain and pain control in children. *Curr Probl Pediatr* 15: 1–67, 1985.

Schneeweis A: *Drug Therapy in Infants and Children with Cardiovascular Disease*. Philadelphia, Lea & Febiger, 1986.

Schou M, Weinstein MR: Problems of lithium maintenance treatment during pregnancy, delivery and lactation. *Agressologie* 21 (Special issue A): 7, 1980.

Shapiro C: Pain in the neonate: Assessment and intervention. *Neonatal Netw* 8: 7–21, 1989.

Snider DE, Powell KE: Should women taking antituberculosis drugs breast-feed? *Arch Intern Med* 144: 589–590, 1984.

Sovner R, Orsulak PJ: Excretion of imipramine and desipramine in human breast milk. *Am J Psychiatry* 136: 451, 1979.

Standards and Guidelines for Cardiopulmonary Resuscitation (CPR) and Emergency Cardiac Care (ECC), Part V: Pediatric advanced life support. *JAMA* 225: 2961–2964, 1986.

Standards and Guidelines for Cardiopulmonary Resuscitation (CPR) and Emergency Cardiac Care (ECC), Part VI: Neonatal advanced life support. *JAMA* 255: 2969–2973, 1986.

Steiner E, Villen T, Hallberg M, Rane A: Amphetamine secretion in milk, *Eur J Clin Pharmacol* 27: 123–124, 1984.

Stiehm ER: Intravenous immunoglobulins in neonates and infants: an overview. *Pediatr Infect Dis* 5 (3 suppl): S 217–219, 1986.

Taeusch HW, Yogman MW (eds): *Follow-up Management of the High Risk Infant.* Boston, Little, Brown & Co, 1987.

Tatro DS (ed): *Drug Interaction Facts.* St. Louis, JB Lippincott Co, 1988.

Trissel LA: *ASHP Handbook on Injectable Drugs,* ed 5. Bethesda, MD, American Society of Hospital Pharmacists Inc, 1988.

Tsang RC, Nichols BL (eds): *Nutrition During Infancy.* Philadelphia, Hanley and Belfus Inc, 1988.

Volpe JJ: *Neurology of the Newborn,* ed 2. Philadelphia, WB Saunders Co, 1987.

Wallach JB: *Interpretation of Pediatric Tests.* Boston, Little, Brown & Co, 1983.

Wallach JB: *Interpretation of Diagnostic Tests,* ed 4. Boston, Little, Brown & Co, 1986.

Weisman LE, Fisher GW, Hemming VG, Peck CC: Pharmacokinetics of intravenous immunoglobulin (Sandoglobulin) in neonates. *Pediatr Infect Dis* 5(3 suppl): s185–188, 1986.

Whaley LF, Wong DL: *Nursing Care of Infants and Children,* ed 3. St. Louis, CV Mosby Co, 1987.

Wilkie RA, Bryan MH: Effect of bronchodilators on airway resistance in ventilator-dependent neonates with chronic lung disease. *J Pediatr* 111: 278–282, 1987.

Wilson DM, Baldwin RB, Ariagno RL: Randomized, placebo-controlled trial of effects of dexamethasone on hypothalamic-pituitary-adrenal axis in preterm infants. *J Pediatr* 113: 764–768, 1988.

Yaffe SJ (ed): *Pediatric Pharmacology, Therapeutic Principles in Practice.* New York, Grune & Stratton Inc, 1980.

Yeh TF (ed): *Drug Therapy in the Neonate and Small Infant.* Chicago, Year Book Medical Publishers, 1985.

Yoder MC, Polin RA: Immunotherapy of neonatal septicemia. *Pediatr Clin North Am* 33: 481–501, 1986.

Young TE, Mangum OB: *Neofax: A Manual of Drugs Used in Neonatal Care.* Columbus, OH, Ross Laboratories, 1988.

Zenk KE: Neonatal cardiovascular drug dosage recommendations. *Periscope* (Newsletter of the California Perinatal Association) Spring 1986.